SELF-ASSESSMENT IN
PSYCHIATRY

SELF-ASSESSMENT IN
PSYCHIATRY

ROGER FARMER
MB, BCh, MRCP, MRCPsych
Lecturer in Psychiatry,
St. Mary's Hospital Medical School,
University of London
Formerly Senior Registrar in Psychiatry,
University Hospital of South Manchester

BLACKWELL
SCIENTIFIC PUBLICATIONS
OXFORD LONDON EDINBURGH
BOSTON MELBOURNE

© 1984 by
Blackwell Scientific Publications
Editorial offices:
Osney Mead, Oxford, OX2 0EL
8 John Street, London, WC1N 2ES
9 Forrest Road, Edinburgh, EH1 2QH
52 Beacon Street, Boston
  Massachusetts 02108, USA
706 Cowper Street, Palo Alto
  California 94301, USA
99 Barry Street, Carlton
  Victoria 3053, Australia

All rights reserved. No part of this
publication may be reproduced, stored
in a retrieval system, or transmitted,
in any form or by any means,
electronic, mechanical, photocopying,
recording or otherwise
without the prior permission of
the copyright owner

First published 1984

Photoset by Enset Ltd,
Midsomer Norton, Bath, Avon
and printed and bound
in Great Britain by
Biddles Ltd,
Guildford and King's Lynn

DISTRIBUTORS

USA
  Blackwell Mosby Book Distributors
  11830 Westline Industrial Drive
  St Louis, Missouri 63141

Canada
  Blackwell Mosby Book Distributors
  120 Melford Drive, Scarborough
  Ontario, M1B 2X4

Australia
  Blackwell Scientific Book Distributors
  31 Advantage Road, Highett
  Victoria 3190

British Library
Cataloguing in Publication Data

Farmer, Roger
  Self-assessment in psychiatry.
  1. Psychiatry—Problems, exercises,
  etc.
  I. Title
  616.89'0076   RC457

ISBN 0-632-01146-7

Contents

	Preface, vi
	The Multiple Choice Question, vii
1–6	The History of Psychiatry, 1
7–12	Research Methodology, 11
13–26	Phenomenology, 15
27–44	Schizophrenia, 25
45–58	Affective Disorders, 43
59–63	Suicide and Deliberate Self-Poisoning or Self-Injury, 59
64–78	Neurosis and Personality Disorder, 65
79–94	Alcoholism, 83
95–103	Drug Dependence, 97
104–107	Sexual Dysfunction, 103
108–121	Organic Psychiatry, 107
122–127	Psychogeriatrics, 121
128–136	Child Psychiatry, 127
137–149	Mental Retardation, 137
150–165	Forensic Psychiatry, 149
166–169	Transcultural Psychiatry, 161
170–188	Physical Methods of Treatment, 165
189–200	Psychological Methods of Treatment, 185

Preface

Revision for examinations can be a lengthy and laborious task. Unfortunately there are no 'magic' shortcuts to spending the time needed studying textbooks and journals. It is very easy, however, to become immersed in a few selected topics and to lose sight of the gaps in your knowledge. It is also surprisingly easy to underestimate what you *do* know and to feel you 'know nothing' as the examination date approaches. Regular self-assessment can help to avoid both these pitfalls. It can expose areas of ignorance but also give confidence by demonstrating areas of relative strength!

This book aims to make revision more enjoyable and to encourage efficient use of limited time. It is intended primarily for those studying for the MRCPsych (Part 2) Membership Examination. More senior psychiatrists may find it of value for teaching purposes and certain questions may be suitable for medical students.

For the examination candidate, in addition to enabling self-assessment, the book should help familiarize him or her with the multiple choice format of question. Unfamiliarity with this style of question can 'throw' even the most knowledgeable of candidates. The book also provides information—probably when the student is at his or her most receptive—immediately after answering a question. As it can be tiresome searching out the relevant information from textbooks or journals (even when page references are given) explanations to nearly all answers are provided. While some explanations are brief and confined to information which the question specifically demands, others are more discursive and include related material. Most students seem to revise piecemeal by subject, so the book is divided into chapters by topic. Suggestions for further reading are offered at the end of each chapter.

I wish to thank Dr D.A.W. Johnson who kindly reviewed a sample of the questions, Marion Philbin for her secretarial assistance, Richard Zorab of Blackwell Scientific Publications for his advice and encouragement, and last but not least my wife—herself a psychiatrist—whose suggestions and support were invaluable.

1984   R.F.

The Multiple Choice Question

'When you have to make a choice and don't make it, that is in itself a choice'

William James

The multiple choice question (MCQ) is now extensively used in examinations. Its advantages lie in its objectivity and the expedience with which results can be analysed.

MCQs test primarily factual knowledge. The format does not lend itself so readily to the assessment of clinical judgment or reasoning skills although some suitably structured questions may have this capability.

Most of the questions in this book are of the *multiple true-false* variety (which is employed in the MRCPsych Membership Examination). Each of these questions consists of a 'stem' followed by several (usually five) items or statements, any number of which may be correct. Each item should be read as a single statement and answered on its own merits. Each statement must be answered as 'True', 'False' or 'Don't know'. In most examinations a penalty marking system is adopted whereby marks are deducted for incorrect answers. In the MRCPsych Membership Examination as much is deducted for an incorrect response as is awarded for a correct one. No marks are given for 'Don't know'; the candidate may assume this is not the correct answer!

Certain information is more readily tested by means of *multiple choice association* questions and a number of these are included. For each numbered word or phrase the most appropriate lettered entity should be selected. In this book each numerical entity has a different lettered equivalent.

Certain adjectives have now rather stereotyped meanings in MCQs. A *characteristic* or *typical* feature is one which occurs sufficiently often in a condition to be of diagnostic significance and whose absence would put the diagnosis in doubt. A *recognized* feature is one which has been reported as occurring in the condition (but which is not necessarily characteristic of it). *Pathognomonic* or *specific* features occur exclusively in the named condition.

In the examination

Allot your time carefully. For instance, if there are 60 questions (each with five parts) to be answered in two hours—as there are in the MRCPsych Membership Examination—this allows two minutes per question. Candidates must ensure they go through the paper at this rate or preferably faster to allow time for reconsideration of answers or to return to difficult questions at the end. Take extra care to mark answers on the answer sheet in the appropriate boxes! Some people prefer to first note their answers on the question paper and later transfer them to the answer sheet. This practice, however, may increase the risk of marking the answers down incorrectly, particularly if poor budgeting of time has left insufficient time for this at the end.

The penalty marking system aims to discourage guessing. Where candidates have absolutely no idea what the correct answer to a question is, a 'Don't know' response seems sensible. Well-prepared candidates, however, approach most questions possessing some relevant knowledge, even if certainty is lacking as to what the correct answer is, and intelligent, educated guessing might be expected to boost the total score.

Remember that the knowledge a question demands will most likely be the generally accepted version of 'the truth'. If you have some special knowledge of a topic, perhaps from personal research, which is at variance with the most prevalent viewpoint, this is the time to swallow your pride!

Further reading

Anderson J. (1982) *The Multiple Choice Question in Medicine*. 2nd edn. London, Pitman.
Lennox B. (1983) Editorial. Even better MCQ books? *Med. Educ.* **17**, 1–2.
Trethowan W.H. (1978) Multiple choice examinations in psychiatry. In Gaind R.N. & Hudson B.L. (eds) *Current Themes in Psychiatry*. pp. 210–18. London, Macmillan Press.

The History of Psychiatry

1   The following were humane reformers:
    A   William Tuke
    B   Benjamin Rush
    C   John Conolly
    D   Philippe Pinel
    E   Thomas Monro

2   Match each of the following names (A–E) with the illness (1–5) he described:
    A   Pick
    B   Hecker
    C   Bleuler
    D   Morel
    E   Kahlbaum

    1   schizophrenia
    2   catatonia
    3   hebephrenia
    4   *démence précoce*
    5   simplex syndrome

1 A C D

In England during the 18th century, patients were confined in Asylums and Private Madhouses, frequently under brutal, degrading conditions. Mechanical restraint was often practised using strait jackets, handcuffs or arm and leg irons. Virtual immobilization could be achieved by the use of the 'tranquillizing chair', in which a hooded patient could be strapped and manacled. This was an invention of the American physician, Benjamin Rush. At the Bethlem Hospital in London succeeding generations of the Monro family carried on treatment practices which included bleeding, purging, vomiting and cupping.

The evidence of a Parliamentary Committee on Madhouses in 1815 added impetus to a movement for humane reform begun at the end of the 18th century and was exemplified by the founding of the Retreat outside York by William Tuke in 1796. Here a system of care based on the tenets of the Quaker religion was practised. In France, Philippe Pinel was responsible for the unchaining of lunatics, first in the Bicêtre in 1793 and later in the Salpêtrière. Conolly was the first to reduce restraint to a minimum in a large County Asylum in England—in 1839 in the Middlesex County Asylum at Hanwell, which had 800 patients.

2 A5 B3 C1 D4 E2

Kraepelin combined the syndromes of *démence précoce*, catatonia (or tension insanity), hebephrenia and dementia paranoides into a group called 'psychological degeneration processes' in 1893. Later, in 1899, he referred to this group as dementia praecox.

'Schizophrenia' is a term introduced by Bleuler in 1911. He considered that a complete *restitutio ad integrum* did not occur from this condition.

Hamilton M. (ed.) (1976) *Fish's Schizophrenia.* p. 1. Bristol, John Wright & Sons.

3 Match each of the following books (A–E) with the person or persons (1–5) who wrote them:
   A *Treatment of the Insane Without Mechanical Restraint*
   B *Anatomy of Melancholy*
   C *Traité Médico-Philosophique sur Aliénation Mentale*
   D *A Description of the Retreat*
   E *Malleus Maleficarum*

   1 Samuel Tuke
   2 Sprenger and Kraemer
   3 Robert Burton
   4 Philippe Pinel
   5 John Conolly

3 A5 B3 C4 D1 E2

In Europe (and North America), until the mid 18th century, a widespread explanation of social deviancy was that it resulted from demoniacal possession. Two Dominican brothers, Sprenger and Kraemer, in 1489 set out for Inquisitors the tenets of witch-hunting in a book entitled *Malleus Maleficarum—The Witches' Hammer*. Status of 'possession' and methods of detection were described.

Robert Burton's *Anatomy of Melancholy* in 1628 set out views which were less extreme but which nevertheless equated lunacy with moral defect. Treatments such as cautery, blistering and bleeding were advocated.

The 19th century saw less restraint and confinement implemented in the care of the mentally disturbed. Samuel Tuke (the founder's grandson) in *A Description of the Retreat*, published 1813, detailed the precepts and methods of the Retreat for Quakers outside York. The philosophy of care of Pinel and Conolly was similar.

Conolly J. (1856) *Treatment of the Insane Without Mechanical Restraint*. Reprinted 1973. London, Dawson & Sons.

Tuke S. (1813) *A Description of the Retreat*. Reprinted 1964. London, Dawson & Sons.

4 Link each of the following treatments (A–E) with the most appropriate person or persons (1–5):
   A lithium
   B electroconvulsive therapy
   C chlorpromazine
   D insulin therapy
   E convulsive therapy
   F psychosurgery

   1 Cerletti and Bini
   2 Delay and Deniker
   3 Moniz
   4 Meduna
   5 Sakel
   6 Arfvedson

4 A6 B1 C2 D5 E4 F3

In 1927 Manfred Sakel in Vienna induced hypoglycaemic coma in schizophrenics by injecting insulin and claimed beneficial effects. At a time when sedation and custodial care were the only alternatives for such patients, the practice spread. Ackner later demonstrated that insulin coma had no specific efficacy and it is likely that the results obtained with *insulin therapy* were attributable to non-specific factors such as selection of good prognosis cases and special nursing care.

Meduna's induction of seizures in schizophrenics in 1933 was based on the premise (now known to be incorrect) that schizophrenia and epilepsy were incompatible. He initially used camphor oil and later cardiazol to induce convulsions. It became apparent that while the results in schizophrenia were disappointing it was often an effective treatment in depression. Cerletti and Bini in 1938 introduced *electroconvulsive therapy*—a more convenient and safer method.

Following Jacobsen and Fulton's results of how frustrational responses in chimpanzees could be modified by frontal lobe surgery, Moniz in 1936 applied *psychosurgery* to psychiatric patients.

Charpentier synthesized *chlorpromazine*. Delay and Deniker in 1952 confirmed suggestions of its tranquillizing properties. It was marketed under the trade name 'Largactil' because of its large variety of pharmacological actions.

The element *lithium* was discovered by Arfvedson in 1817. Its cardiotoxicity ended earlier therapeutic trials in gout and as a sodium chloride substitute for cardiac patients. However, in 1949 Cade reported beneficial effects of lithium in mania and evidence for this and for a prophylactic effect on recurrent affective disorder was obtained by Schou in clinical trials.

5   Match each of the following names (A–E) with the concept (1–5) he described:
    A   Henderson
    B   Schneider
    C   Pritchard
    D   Pinel
    E   Koch

    1   moral insanity
    2   creative psychopathy
    3   psychopathic inferiority
    4   mania without confusion
    5   psychopathic personalities

5 A2 B5 C1 D4 E3
The concept of *psychopathy* remains one unreliably used by psychiatrists.

Pinel, in 1801, was one of the first to describe *manie sans délire (mania without confusion)*. The condition was one of emotional and volitional disturbance without any intellectual abnormality. Benjamin Rush, in 1812, considered *moral derangement* was present in such cases and that medical treatment was appropriate. In 1835, Pritchard in England described *moral insanity* as a form of madness without intellectual impairment or any psychotic features. Koch, in 1891, introduced the terms *psychopath, psychopathic inferior* and *constitutional inferior*.

Schneider, in using the term *psychopathic personality*, included what is now regarded as neurosis and personality disorder. 'Psychopathic personalities' were abnormal personalities who either suffered themselves or caused society to suffer; the former corresponding roughly to our present day concept of neurosis and the latter to sociopathic personality disorder.

In 1937 Henderson described three main types of psychopath—the inadequate, the aggressive and the creative. Of these the last has probably had the least impact on nosology.

Thorley A. & Stern R. (1979) Origins of the concept of psychopathic personality. In Hill P., Murray R. & Thorley A. (eds) *Essentials of Postgraduate Psychiatry*. pp. 231–4. London, Academic Press.

6 Match each of the following names (A−E) with the concept (1−5) with which he is associated:
   A Jackson
   B Meyer
   C Jaspers
   D Kretschmer
   E Kraepelin

   1 *der sensitive Beziehungswahn*
   2 separation of dementia praecox from manic-depressive insanity
   3 stratification of mental function
   4 understandability
   5 psychobiology

6 A3 B5 C4 D1 E2
Having described *dementia praecox*, Kraepelin (1856–1926) distinguished it from manic-depressive insanity on the grounds of prognosis. In his view the former usually, but not invariably, had a progressive course while the latter was characterized by remissions between episodes of illness.

Kretschmer (1888–1964) described *der sensitive Beziehungswahn* (delusions of self-reference in a sensitive person). After meticulously tracing out the past histories of certain individuals with paranoid psychosis he concluded that their delusions were the understandable outcome of their experiences.

The criterion *understandability* of symptoms in psychiatry was introduced by Jaspers (1883–1969). Where symptoms could not be understood as arising from the personality, he hypothesized a 'psychic process'; where they could, he considered the condition a personality 'development'.

Adolf Meyer (1866–1950) founded a school of thought called *'psychobiology'* based on a synthesis of Freudian (psychoanalytical) theory and more traditional psychiatry. He regarded mental illness as the reaction of the personality to life stress. Emphasis was placed on tracing a person's total life experience in order to understand their unique clinical presentation.

Hughlings Jackson (1834–1911) conceptualized the central nervous system as having different levels of function, release of lower level functions occurring as the result of disturbance at a higher level.

Kretschmer E. (1974) Der sensitive Beziehungswahn. Selected sections in Hirsch S.R. & Shepherd M. (eds) *Themes and Variations in European Psychiatry*. p. 153. Bristol, John Wright & Sons.

Further reading

Ackerknecht E.H. (1959) *A Short History of Psychiatry*, trans. by Wolff S. London, Hafner Publishing Company.
Hunter R. & MacAlpine I. (1963) *Three Hundred Years of Psychiatry 1535–1860*. London, Oxford University Press.
Lader M. & Allderidge P. (1976) *The History of British Psychiatry 1700 to the Present*. London, SK & F Publications.

Research Methodology

7 Reliability of an instrument
A is high if ratings of the same material by different raters using that instrument are similar
B concerns the repeatability of its measurement
C means it measures what it is intended to
D is high if its measurements accord with those of another instrument supposed to have the same function
E is concerned with the accuracy of its measurements

8 A placebo in a clinical trial
A should be given with as much confidence as the 'active' drug
B is pharmacologically inert
C should be identical in appearance to the drug being studied
D has no effects
E is best administered by someone who is unaware of the tablet's contents

9 Placebo effects
A bear no relation to tablet size
B are more likely in older people
C are influenced by the status of the therapist
D include headache
E are stronger in introverts

7 A B E

Reliability of a measuring instrument is the degree to which there is repeatability of its scores and is therefore concerned with the accuracy or precision of the measurement.

Validity, on the other hand, is the extent to which an instrument measures what it purports to measure.

It follows that an instrument may be reliable while not necessarily valid in its measurements.

8 A B C E

A placebo is a pharmacologically inert substance which may, however, exert effects through psychological mechanisms such as suggestion. It may be used as a control in studies to determine the efficacy of medicines, in which case the placebo should have an identical appearance to the medicinal substance and should be administered with equal enthusiasm and confidence. This is best fulfilled under double-blind conditions.

In practice, however, the placebo may be distinguishable by therapist or patient because it lacks side-effects specifically associated with the 'active' drug. For this reason, substances with atropine-like properties have been used as controls in some clinical trials of anti-depressant drugs.

9 C D

Placebo effects are influenced by the status of the therapist, his attitude towards the treatment and the expectations of the patient. Hence a beneficial outcome may be partly due to a well-respected doctor showing enthusiasm and confidence in the treatment.

The appearance and quality of tablets may also be influential. For instance, very small or very large tablets appear to exert more effect than medium-sized ones.

Placebo reactors (those who respond to placebos) tend to be younger patients, of lower intelligence, sociable and outgoing, but more anxious in the treatment setting. Placebos may be more effective in acute conditions including headache, post-operative pain and motion sickness. Adverse side-effects have been reported with placebos, such as drowsiness, nausea and headache.

Silverstone T. & Turner P. (1978) *Drug Treatment in Psychiatry*. pp. 76–80. London, Routledge & Kegan Paul.

10 In a double-blind trial comparing two drugs
A the experimenter is unable to assess the dependent variable
B both experimenter and subject know what the independent variable is for that subject
C the experimenter is unaware of which drug the subject receives
D the drugs are the dependent variable
E the subject does not know which drug he is taking

11 The Hawthorne effect refers to
A the adverse effects of the drug being studied
B a patient's performance improving with practice
C the presence of researchers being a confounding variable
D the effect of the subject on the researcher
E subjects showing improved performance when studied

12 Match each of the following statements (A–F) with the rating scale source of error (1–6) it describes:

Some responders tend to
A make a moderate rather than an extreme rating
B give an incorrect response rather than divulge personal information
C either agree or disagree excessively with the propositions
D be influenced in making a response by the adjoining ratings
E choose the acceptable rather than the true response
F make a response compatible with a concept such as diagnosis suggested by previous responses

1 response set
2 defensiveness
3 social desirability
4 bias towards the middle
5 halo effect
6 proximity

10 C E

In any study the *independent variable* is the condition manipulated by the experimenter (e.g. the drug administered to the subject) while the *dependent variable* is the effect of the independent variable (e.g. therapeutic or adverse drug effects).

In a *single-blind* trial only the subject is unaware of the independent variable applicable to him (e.g. which drug he is receiving); however, in a *double-blind* study both experimenter and subject are kept blind to this.

11 C E

This effect is particularly likely to occur when patients who have been relatively ignored previously are suddenly shown interest and attention as subjects of research.

B is an example of *practice effect* whereby if successive assessments are made a subject's performance may alter; for instance, it may improve because he feels less anxious or his skill in carrying out a task has increased with practice, or it may deteriorate because the task has become tedious.

12 A4 B2 C1 D6 E3 F5

Social desirability and *defensiveness* are potential sources of error specific to self-report questionnaires (i.e. those filled in by the patient himself) while *proximity* and *halo effect* apply only to observer-rated schedules (i.e. those filled in about the patient by someone else such as a doctor, a nurse or even a relative). *Response set* and *bias towards the middle* are sources of error common to both kinds of instrument. Ways have been devised of reducing such errors such as the incorporation of a Lie Scale in the Eysenck Personality Inventory intended to detect those whose responses are untrue in order to be defensive or socially desirable.

Further reading

Mann A. & Murray R. (1979) Measurement in psychiatry. In Hill P., Murray R. & Thorley A. (eds) *Essentials of Postgraduate Psychiatry.* pp. 77–98. London, Academic Press.

Sainsbury P. & Kreitman N. (eds) (1975) *Methods of Psychiatric Research. An Introduction for Clinical Psychiatrists.* Oxford, Oxford University Press.

Phenomenology

13 The following are passivity experiences:
   A thought block
   B obsessional rituals
   C pressured speech
   D 'made' acts
   E echopraxia

14 The following are recognized features of the Ganser syndrome:
   A approximate answers
   B delusions of persecution
   C *vorbeireden*
   D hallucinations
   E depressed mood

15 The following are true of delusions:
   A they are abnormal beliefs
   B their content is often fantastic
   C the beliefs may be shared by those of similar cultural background
   D they are unshakeable by reason
   E the beliefs are invariably false

16 The following are illusions:
   A micropsia
   B *écho de pensées*
   C perceptions without an external stimulus
   D formication
   E false assessments of correct perceptions

13 D

Patients with passivity experiences believe that some external force is influencing their thoughts, feelings or actions—hence, for example, 'made' acts.

While thought insertion and thought withdrawal are related phenomena, thought block refers simply to the experience of a sudden stopping of thoughts (which may not be attributed to anything in particular by the patient).

As with thought block, patients with obsessional rituals, pressured speech or echopraxia do not necessarily have an experience of some external control or influence.

14 A C D

The Ganser syndrome has four recognized clinical features: the approximate answer, clouding of consciousness, somatic conversion and hallucinations. The approximate answer is a response which is incorrect, but nevertheless suggestive that the correct answer exists in the patient's mind, e.g. an answer that a horse has five legs or that 2+2 is 5. This has also been referred to as *vorbeireden* or talking past the point.

Delusions of persecution and depressed mood are not recognized features.

15 A B D

Delusions are abnormal beliefs, which are incorrigible, i.e. unamenable to reason, idiosyncratic, i.e. not shared by people of the same cultural background, often preoccupying and often absurd. A delusional belief may rarely be true; this is probably most commonly encountered in morbid jealousy.

16 A

Illusions are incorrect perceptions of real objects and an example is micropsia (seeing objects as smaller than they actually are). Perceptions in the absence of an external stimulus are termed *hallucinations*. Examples are *écho de pensées* and formication, which take the form of hearing one's own thoughts spoken aloud and a sensation of animals crawling over one's body, respectively. Making an incorrect deduction from a correct perception is referred to as *misinterpretation*.

17 The following are true of obsessional thoughts:
A they are frequently resisted
B they support a diagnosis of schizophrenia
C aggressive themes frequently lead to actual harm occurring
D they are typically experienced as implanted from the outside
E the content may be concerned with contamination

18 The following statements concerning de Clérambault's syndrome are true:
A the person who is the object of the delusional belief is freqeuntly of a higher social status than the patient
B a patient, usually a man, has a delusional belief that someone is in love with him
C the patient often craves for a sexual relationship
D it has been referred to as 'erotomania'
E the person selected is often much older than the patient

19 The following statements concerning schizophrenic formal thought disorder are true:
A Bannister suggested that the clinical features result from a loose and inconsistent construct system
B it is a disorder of conceptual thinking
C Cameron drew attention to overinclusiveness
D interpenetration of themes may be a feature
E decreased redundancy of words occurs

17 A E

In definitions of obsessional thoughts emphasis has been placed variously on a subjective sense of compulsion, resistance to them and recognition of their senseless nature. Resistance is typically at the expense of mounting anxiety. While the subject with thought insertion experiences foreign thoughts intruding into his mind, obsessional thoughts are recognized as subjective, i.e. as his own thoughts.

Common themes concern contamination, blasphemy, sex and aggression; however, aggressive themes are rarely translated into violence.

Obsessional phenomena are not of diagnostic value in schizophrenia.

18 A C D E

In de Clérambault's syndrome the patient, who is generally a *woman*, has a delusional belief that a man is in love with her. This belief is not typically founded on platonic love and the patient often desires a sexual relationship. The person selected, i.e. the object of the belief, is likely to be unattainable, on account of, for example, his age, higher social status, being already married or being a public figure.

19 A B C D E

Schizophrenic formal thought disorder (SFTD) is a disorder of conceptual or abstract thinking. A similar disorder of thought form can occur in organic brain disease.

Redundancy in this context refers to the predictability of a word occurring in speech. In SFTD, as expressed in speech, words are less easily predicted and hence redundancy is less.

Bannister has postulated that the clinical features of SFTD result from a loose and inconsistent construct system. He used a Repertory Grid test derived from Kelly's Personal Construct Theory.

Cameron called the vague, imprecise mode of thinking in schizophrenia 'asyndetic' and described interpenetration and overinclusiveness in such thinking.

20 **The following are true of morbid jealousy:**
   A   alcoholism is a primary cause in the majority of cases
   B   the Othello syndrome is an eponymous title
   C   it occurs in schizophrenia
   D   a dominant theme is preoccupation with the partner's sexual unfaithfulness
   E   there is an association with overt homosexuality

21 **The following are true of delusional mood:**
   A   it may be shared by people of the same religious background
   B   the appearance of a sudden delusional idea (autochthonous delusion) may bring relief
   C   it is a Schneiderian first rank symptom
   D   a sudden delusional idea (autochthonous delusion) may occur, arising understandably from the mood
   E   it is a variety of primary delusion

20 B C D
Morbid jealousy is probably best viewed as a descriptive term rather than as a diagnosis. The central theme is a preoccupation with the partner's infidelity. It may be a symptom of various psychiatric conditions, including schizophrenia. Surveys suggest that between one-third and one-half of morbidly jealous patients suffer from psychotic disorders, about the same proportion from neuroses and personality disorders, while alcoholism is a primary diagnosis in less than 7 per cent of cases. Although alcoholism frequently aggravates pre-existing symptoms and may lead to violence, it is seldom a primary cause of morbid jealousy.

Although Freud suggested that unconscious homosexual feelings play a part in all jealousy, an association between overt homosexuality and morbid jealousy has not been demonstrated.

Cobb J. (1979) Morbid jealousy. *Br. J. Hosp. Med.* **21**, 511–18.
Shepherd M. (1961) Morbid jealousy, some clinical and social aspects of a psychiatric symptom. *J. Ment. Sci.* **107**, 687.

21 B E
Unlike secondary delusions, primary delusions cannot be understood as arising from some other psychological symptom. Delusional mood, the sudden delusional idea and delusional perception are all varieties of primary delusion, but Schneider included only delusional perception as a first rank symptom in diagnosing schizophrenia. In delusional mood the patient usually feels tense and bewildered. A primary delusion may then appear as a sudden delusional idea or delusional perception often bringing a sense of relief.

A delusion is not shared by people of the same religious, educational or cultural background (see Question 15).

22 Complex visual hallucinations occur in
  A paranoid schizophrenia
  B phobic neurosis
  C occipital epileptic seizures
  D delirium tremens
  E centrencephalic epilepsy

23 Hallucinations
  A are under voluntary control
  B were considered by Jaspers to be a special kind of imagery
  C can sometimes be discriminated by patients from actual perceptions
  D are experienced as emanating from the mind
  E are distortions of real perceptions

24 The Capgras phenomenon
  A usually accompanies a paranoid psychosis
  B typically involves a patient believing that a person unrelated to him has been replaced by a double
  C is an example of a delusion
  D can occur at any time during the course of the psychosis
  E only occurs in schizophrenia

Phenomenology: Answers

22 A D

Visual hallucinations may occur in epilepsy as part of the aura. When seizures originate within the occipital lobe—*occipital seizures*—complex hallucinations which convey meaning do not occur, although simple hallucinations such as flashes of light or field defects such as hemianopias may be experienced.

In *centrencephalic epilepsy* the site of origin of the fit is subcortical and a generalized convulsion occurs without any preceding aura.

(A distinction should be drawn between 'auras' and 'prodromata'. The latter build up gradually over hours or days and consist of mood changes such as apprehension or irritability, headaches, gastrointestinal symptoms and autonomic changes such as flushing or pallor.)

Complex visual hallucinations may occur in *delirium tremens* or *paranoid schizophrenia*. Hallucinations in acute organic reactions such as delirium tremens are usually visual. In paranoid schizophrenia, however, auditory hallucinations are more typical.

Hallucinations do not occur in *phobic neuroses*.

23 C

According to Jaspers, *hallucinations* are false perceptions and distinct from *pseudohallucinations*, which he considered to be a form of mental imagery and hence experienced as arising from the mind. Both hallucinations and pseudohallucinations are involuntary phenomena. Patients frequently have little difficulty in distinguishing between hallucinations and real perceptions, particularly in the chronic stages of psychosis.

Distortions of real perceptions are generally termed illusions (see Question 16).

24 A C D

The Capgras phenomenon is a delusion that a person usually closely related to the patient has been replaced by an exact double. Its occurrence is rare. In married patients the spouse is nearly always the person selected. It usually accompanies a paranoid psychosis, either of the schizophrenic or affective type, and can occur at any time during the course of the illness.

25 The following are true of schizophrenic formal thought disorder:
A clang association is a characteristic feature
B Goldstein considered impairment of abstract thinking to be partly responsible
C Kurt Schneider described derailment and drivelling
D an association between one idea and the next may not be apparent
E confabulation is a recognized feature

26 The following are recognized catatonic signs:
A echopraxia
B cataplexy
C negativism
D *Schnauzkrampf*
E cleaning rituals

25 B D

Eugen Bleuler considered that the basic abnormality in schizophrenic formal thought disorder (SFTD) was a disorder of association, so that the connection between one theme and the next may not be obvious.

Goldstein drew attention to concrete thinking in schizophrenics while *Carl* Schneider described the following kinds of SFTD: fusion, derailment, omission, drivelling and substitution (Kurt is the Schneider of 'first rank symptoms' fame).

Clang association describes verbal association by rhyme, which occurs characteristically in flight of ideas in hypomania, not SFTD.

Confabulation is the fabrication of false memories and, while it may occur in dysmnesic patients, it is not a recognized feature of schizophrenics.

26 A C D

While *catalepsy* is a catatonic sign, *cataplexy* is not, and refers to sudden attacks of muscle weakness and hypotonia, which occur as part of the narcolepsy syndrome, along with hypnagogic hallucinations and sleep paralysis.

Catalepsy refers to preservation by the patient of any posture in which he is placed, usually associated with waxy rigidity (or *flexibilitas cerea*).

Cleaning rituals are a manifestation of obsessional neurosis and are not a recognized catatonic sign.

Further reading

Clare A. (1980) The diagnostic process. In Clare A. (ed.) *Psychiatry in Dissent: Controversial Issues in Thought and Practice.* 2nd edn. pp. 76–119. London, Tavistock Publications.

Enoch M.D. & Trethowan W.H. (1979) *Uncommon Psychiatric Syndromes.* 2nd edn. Bristol, John Wright & Sons.

Hamilton M. (ed.) (1974) *Fish's Clinical Psychopathology.* Bristol, John Wright & Sons.

Hirsch S.R. & Shepherd M. (1974) *Themes and Variations in European Psychiatry.* Bristol, John Wright & Sons.

Jaspers K. (1959) *General Psychopathology.* 7th edn. Trans. Hoenig J. & Hamilton M. Manchester, Manchester University Press.

Kraupl Taylor F. (1979) *Psychopathology: Its Causes and Symptoms.* Sunbury, Quatermaine.

Mullen P. (1979) The phenomenology of disordered mental function. In Hill P., Murray R. & Thorley A. (ed.) *Essentials of Postgraduate Psychiatry.* pp. 25–54. London, Academic Press.

Shepherd M. & Zangwill O.L. (eds) (1983) *Handbook of Psychiatry 1. General Psychopathology.* Cambridge, Cambridge University Press.

Schizophrenia

27 Brown and Birley (1968), in looking at the onset of schizophrenic symptoms, found there was a more frequent than expected occurrence of life events
   A before admission if events independent of illness were considered
   B in the three weeks before admission
   C before admission which could be wholly accounted for by the patient's effort after meaning
   D before admission only if 'severe' events were considered
   E none of the above

28 The following are Schneiderian first rank symptoms:
   A delusional mood
   B *Gedankenlautwerden*
   C hallucinatory voices talking to the patient
   D a delusion of having one's thoughts read
   E thought insertion

27 A B

Brown and Birley (1968) suggested that a higher than expected frequency of life events occurred in the three weeks before admission with schizophrenic symptoms. The life events in question were not necessarily severely threatening.

A possible objection to establishing an aetiological link between life events and illness such as schizophrenia is that events could have been related to the insidious onset of the illness. For instance, the break-up of a relationship could have been due to an illness-related change in the subject's behaviour. In an attempt to overcome this objection, Brown classifies events which were outside the subject's control as 'independent' and assesses them separately from 'possibly independent' and illness-related events.

It is possible that a subject's assessment of past events will be influenced by his present psychiatric condition. For instance, in an 'effort after meaning' a depressed person may view his past in a more unfortunate light. Brown attempts to avoid such retrospective falsification. Raters are presented with descriptions of events but are blind to the subject's mental state and reporting of the event's severity.

Brown G.W. & Birley J.L.T. (1968) Crises and life changes and the onset of schizophrenia. *J. Health Soc. Behav.* **9**, 203–14.

Brown G.W. & Harris T. (1978) *Social Origins of Depression: A Study of Psychiatric Disorder in Women.* London, Tavistock Publications.

Tennant C., Bebbington P. & Hurry J. (1981) The role of life events in depressive illness: is there a substantial causal relation? *Psychol. Med.* **1**, 379–89.

28 B E

Schneider described 'symptoms of the first rank', each of which he considered diagnostic of schizophrenia in the absence of coarse brain disease. They consist of:
1 Auditory hallucinations of three kinds:
   (a) voices repeating the patient's thoughts out loud (thought echo, in German *Gedankenlautwerden*, or in French *écho de pensées*)
   (b) voices discussing or arguing about the patient, referring to him in the third person
   (c) voices commenting on the patient's thoughts or behaviour, often as a running commentary.
2 Delusional perception.
3 Thought insertion, thought withdrawal or thought broadcast.
4 Passivity experiences—'made' acts, impulses or feelings.
5 Somatic passivity—the experience that bodily sensations are produced by outside agencies.

Kendell R.E. (1972) Schizophrenia: the remedy for diagnostic confusion. *Br. J. Hosp. Med.* **8**, 383–90.

Mellor C.S. (1970) First rank symptoms of schizophrenia. *Br. J. Psychiat.* **117**, 15.

29 Pair each of the following conditions (A–E) with the person or persons who named it (1–5):
A schizo-affective psychosis
B pseudoneurotic schizophrenia
C latent schizophrenia
D schizophreniform psychosis
E oneirophrenia

1 Hoch and Polatin
2 Langfeldt
3 Kasanin
4 Mayer-Gross
5 Bleuler

30 The following statements concerning concordance rate in twin studies are true:
A the pairwise method involves counting each concordant pair (twinship) twice
B the probandwise rate for schizophrenia in monozygotic twins is about 30 per cent
C probandwise method yields an estimate of heritability similar to that derived from family studies
D the pairwise method gives numerically higher values for the concordance than the probandwise method
E the probandwise rate for schizophrenia in dizygotic twins is approximately 15 per cent

29 A3 B1 C5 D2 E4

Kasanin applied the term *schizo-affective* to cases of acute psychosis with a mixture of schizophrenic and affective symptoms.

Langfeldt described rather similar patients and coined the term *schizophreniform psychosis*. He emphasized the condition's good prognosis and separated such cases from 'nuclear' or 'process' schizophrenia.

In *pseudoneurotic schizophrenia* described by Hoch and Polatin anxiety occurs. Symptoms of different neurotic illnesses may be simultaneously present in the same patient as may various sexual deviations. Psychotic episodes may briefly occur.

Mayer-Gross described as *oneroid states* or *oneirophrenia* dream-like psychotic states with scenic hallucinations during which alteration of consciousness may appear to occur.

Bleuler reserved the term *latent schizophrenia* for those subjects with abnormal personalities who had had in his view a once insidious but now inactive schizophrenic illness.

Gunderson J.G. & Singer M.T. (1975) Defining borderline patients: an overview. *Am. J. Psychiat.* **132**, 1–9.

Procci W.R. (1976) Schizo-affective psychosis: fact or fiction? *Arch. Gen. Psychiat.* **33**, 1167–78.

30 C E

Concordance may be estimated in two ways. The percentage of pairs in which both twins are affected (concordant pairs) may be calculated—the *pairwise rate*. Alternatively, each affected twin or proband may be considered and the percentage where the co-twin is also affected estimated—the *probandwise rate*. In the latter method concordant twinships or pairs may be counted twice and therefore the proband method will give higher estimates of concordance than the pairwise method.

In practice the probandwise method gives a reliable estimate of heritability, similar to that estimated from family studies.

When the results of five recent twin studies on schizophrenia were averaged for probandwise concordance rate, the rate for monozygotic twins was 47 per cent and for dizygotic twins 14 per cent (Gottesman and Shields, 1976).

Gottesman I.I. & Shields J. (1976) *Schizophr. Bull.* **2**, 364.

Kreitman N. & Clayton R.M. (1978) Genetic aspects of mental disorder. In Forrest A., Affleck J. & Zealley A. (eds) *Companion to Psychiatric Studies*. pp. 128–59. Edinburgh, Churchill Livingstone.

31 The following statements concerning the epidemiology of schizophrenia are true:
   A   prevalence rate is between 2 and 9 per 1000
   B   incidence rates are highest in the elderly
   C   outside the USA, expectancy or lifetime risk is 2 per cent
   D   age of onset is later in men than women
   E   more schizophrenics are born in the summer than in any other season

32 An individual shares on average 50 per cent of his genes with his
   A   grandfather
   B   monozygotic twin
   C   nephew
   D   daughter
   E   dizygotic twin

31 A

Prevalence, incidence and expectancy are the main indices of morbidity used in epidemiological surveys.

Incidence rates for schizophrenia are highest in young adults and the age of onset tends to be later in women than in men.

Expectancy or *lifetime risk* is an index of morbidity most applicable to the study of chronic progressive illnesses. Modern studies have underlined the variability of outcome in schizophrenia, limiting the validity of this index in schizophrenia research. Most surveys outside the USA have estimated the lifetime risk at under 1 per cent. Estimates in the USA where diagnostic criteria have been broader, have been between 1 and 3 per cent.

There is an increased incidence of schizophrenia in the winter-born. An agent such as a virus, prevalent during the winter months, and causing schizophrenia has been postulated.

Cooper B. (1978) Epidemiology. In Wing J.K. (ed.) *Schizophrenia. Towards a New Synthesis.* pp. 31–52. London, Academic Press.

Hare E. (1982) Epidemiology of schizophrenia. In Wing J.K. & Wing L. (eds) *Handbook of Psychiatry—3.* pp. 42–8. Cambridge, Cambridge University Press.

32 D E

A person will have on average half his genes in common with a first degree relative (parent, full sibling or child) and 25 per cent in common with a second degree relative (uncle, aunt, nephew, niece, grandparent, grandchild or half-sibling).

Monozygotic twins are identical in genotype while dizygotic twins are no more alike than full siblings in respect to their genes.

33 Link each of the following names or pairs of names (A–E) with the most appropriate aetiological concept (1–5):
A Lidz
B Gottesman and Shields
C Fromm-Reichmann
D Slater
E Wynne and Singer

1 polygenic inheritance
2 communication defects and deviances
3 monogenic model of inheritance
4 schizophrenogenic mother
5 marital schism and skew

33 A5 B1 C4 D3 E2

Lidz and his colleagues (1965) described *marital schism and skew*, which appeared, in their numerically limited study, to characterize the parental relationships of female and male schizophrenics respectively. 'Schism' refers to a relationship of hatred with conflict or mutual withdrawal. 'Skew' occurs when one partner, usually the mother, is dominant and demanding while the spouse is ineffectual and compliant.

Frieda Fromm-Reichmann (1948) first used the term *schizophrenogenic mother* and considered such mothers to be dominant and threatening. More systematic studies (e.g. Waring and Ricks, 1965; Gardner, 1967) have found the mothers of schizophrenics to be in contrast shy and inadequate.

Wynne and Singer suggested that the parents of schizophrenics have abnormal modes of communication and were able to predict with impressive accuracy whether or not subjects were schizophrenic by blindly assessing the speech of their parents for *communication defects and deviances* (1963). A study by Hirsch and Leff (1975) failed to replicate these findings.

Slater proposed a *monogenic model* of inheritance whereby the same abnormal gene is responsible for schizophrenia. Gottesman and Shields have suggested that schizophrenia is the result of the combined effect of many genes—a *polygenic model*. *Genetic heterogeneity*, a third model, assumes that schizophrenia consists of different conditions each with a different heredity.

Fromm-Reichmann F. (1948) Notes on the development of treatment of schizophrenics by psychoanalytic psychotherapy. *Psychiatry* **11**, 263–73.
Gardner G.G. (1967) The role of maternal psychopathology in male and female schizophrenics. *J. Consult. Psychol.* **31**, 411–13.
Hirsch S. & Leff J.P. (1975) *Abnormalities in Parents of Schizophrenics*. Maudsley Monograph No. 22. Oxford, Oxford University Press.
Lidz T., Cornelison A.R., Singer M.T., Schafer S. & Fleck S. (1965) The mothers of schizophrenic patients. In Lidz T., Fleck S. & Cornelison A.R. (eds) *Schizophrenia and the Family*. New York, International Universities Press.
Reveley A. & Murray R.M. (1980) The genetic contribution to the functional psychoses. *Br. J. Hosp. Med.* **24**, 166–71.
Waring M. & Ricks D. (1965) Family patterns of children who became adult schizophrenics. *J. Nerv. Ment. Dis.* **140**, 351–64.
Wynne L.C. & Singer M.T. (1963) Thought disorder and family relationships of schizophrenics: II A classification of forms of thinking. *Arch. Gen. Psychiat.* **9**, 199–206.

Schizophrenia: Questions

34 According to Vaughn and Leff (1976), relapse of schizophrenia
A occurred more often if the relative with whom the patient lived made critical comments
B was less likely if a high 'expressed emotion' relative spent more than 35 hours with the patient
C was not affected by neuroleptic medication when the relative showed high 'expressed emotion' (EE)
D was higher in rate during the nine month period studied when the relative exhibited high 'expressed emotion'
E did not occur in the patients studied if neuroleptic medication was given and the relative showed low 'expressed emotion'

35 The following predict good prognosis in schizophrenia:
A insidious onset
B flattening of affect
C family history of affective disorder
D poverty of speech
E history of precipitating factor

34 A D

Vaughn and Leff (1976) replicated findings of Brown *et al.* (1972) that relapse of schizophrenic symptoms in the nine months following discharge from hospital was related to three measures of emotional expression of a key relative—critical comments, hostility and over-involvement.

When data from the two studies were pooled the influences on relapse rate of neuroleptic medication and the amount of face-to-face contact between patient and relative were clarified and may be summarized as follows (nine month relapse rates (Vaughn & Leff, 1976)):

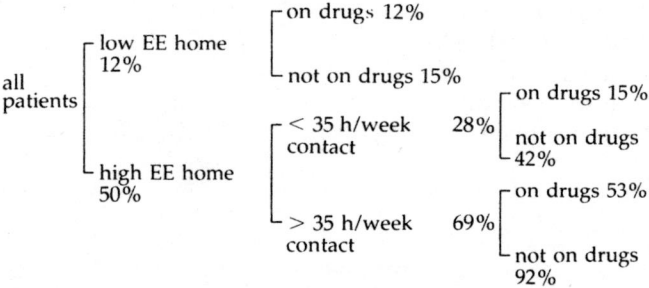

In the high EE relative group if neither protective factor (low face-to-face contact or neuroleptic medication) is present nearly all patients relapse. The presence of one or other protective factor reduces the rate of relapse by about half. If both protective factors are present the rate of relapse is at a low level similar to that in patients from low EE homes.

Brown G.W., Birley J.L.T. & Wing J.L. (1972) The influence of family life on the course of schizophrenic disorders—a replication. *Br. J. Psychiat.* **121**, 241–58.

Vaughn C. & Leff J.P. (1976) The influence of family and social factors on the course of psychiatric illness. *Br. J. Psychiat.* **29**, 125–37.

35 C E

The following are generally held to be predictors of good prognosis in schizophrenia: good premorbid personality, family history of affective disorder, evidence of precipitating factors, acute onset and presence of affective symptoms.

Flattening of affect and poverty of speech are features of chronic schizophrenia.

Myers D.H. (1978) Prognosis of schizophrenia. *Br. J. Hosp. Med.* **20**, 516.

Schizophrenia: Questions

36 The following support the dopamine hypothesis:
A the limbic area of the brain is rich in dopaminergic nerve endings
B amphetamine psychosis
C antipsychotic drugs cause Parkinsonism
D turnover of dopamine is either normal or reduced in schizophrenia
E amphetamines release noradrenaline into the synaptic cleft
F blood prolactin levels in schizophrenic are normal

37 With reference to the social disablement of a schizophrenic patient the following are extrinsic disadvantages:
A adverse personal reactions to impairment
B hallucinations
C secondary handicap
D lack of family support
E institutionalization

36 A B C

The hypothesis that schizophrenia results from an overactive dopamine (DA) system is based on two findings:
1 Amphetamines can produce a syndrome very similar to paranoid schizophrenia (for the effects of amphetamines on transmitter systems see Question 171).
2 The antipsychotic efficacy of neuroleptic drugs correlates with their tendency to cause Parkinsonian symptoms (which are due to functional DA deficiency in the nigrostriatal pathway).

The hypothesized overactivity of the DA system might be due to either increased release of DA into synapses or hypersensitivity of postsynaptic receptors. The following findings in schizophrenia argue against the former possibility:
1 Normal prolactin levels.
2 Normal or reduced DA turnover (assessed by urinary excretion of DA or its metabolites, or estimations of CSF homovanillic acid after probenecid administration).
3 Absence of antipsychotic efficacy of α-methyl-p-tyrosine which inhibits DA synthesis.

Some evidence for receptor hypersensitivity in schizophrenia is offered by postmortem receptor binding studies.

37 D

Three kinds of impairment together constitute the social disablement associated with schizophrenia:
1 Intrinsic impairment (or primary handicap)—disablement due to the symptoms of the illness, such as delusional beliefs, emotional flattening or poverty of speech.
2 Extrinsic disadvantage (or premorbid handicap) such as poor education or lack of social support.
3 Adverse personal reactions (or secondary handicap), an extreme form of which is institutionalization with lack of volition and an apparent satisfaction with life in an institution.

Wing J.K. & Morris B. (eds) (1981) *Handbook of Psychiatric Rehabilitation Practice.* Oxford, Oxford University Press.

Schizophrenia: Questions

38 Typically double-bind communications
A occur in a relaxed setting
B are given by a stranger
C involve two or more conflicting messages
D lead to the recipient escaping from the conflict by laughing it off
E none of the above

39 The following are typical features of chronic schizophrenia:
A delusions of control
B hallucinatory experiences
C poverty of speech
D social withdrawal
E inactivity

40 The following were regarded by Bleuler as primary symptoms of schizophrenia:
A ambivalence
B delusional mood
C emotional flattening
D auditory hallucinations
E loosening of association in thought

41 Dimethyltryptamine (DMT) is
A present in the urine of normal subjects
B psychotomimetic
C an N-methylated derivative of tryptamine
D normally synthesized in the body
E all of the above

38 C

Bateson and others have postulated that receiving double-bind messages as a child might lead to the development of schizophrenia as a means of coping with the intolerable conflict.

Double-bind communications are characteristically given by someone important to the child such as his mother, in a setting of emotional arousal. The social context prevents the child from resolving or escaping from the conflict.

Bateson G., Jackson D.D., Haley J.O. & Weakland J. (1956) Towards a theory of schizophrenia. *Behav. Sci.* **1,** 251–64.

39 C D E

Other characteristic features of chronic schizophrenia are lack of volition, behavioural and cognitive slowing and flattening of affect. Formal thought disorder may also occur in the chronic syndrome.

Schneider's first rank symptoms (see Question 28), which include delusions of control and certain types of auditory hallucinations, tend to characterize acute episodes of the condition.

40 A C E

Delusions, hallucinations and catatonic symptoms were considered by Bleuler to be secondary or accessory symptoms in schizophrenia. Autism (withdrawal) was intermediate in significance, between the primary and secondary groups of symptoms, in Bleuler's system.

41 A B C D E

Findings related to DMT provide a recent thread in the transmethylation hypothesis of schizophrenia. This substance is (like psilocybin) an N-methylated derivative of tryptamine and a potent psychotomimetic agent. It occurs in small amounts in the urine of normal subjects and a biosynthetic pathway exists.

Some, but not all, studies suggest its excretion is increased in the urine of psychotic patients.

Schizophrenia: Questions

42 Unusually high prevalence rates of schizophrenia have been reported in the following groups:
  A the Tamils of southern India
  B Norwegian emigrants to America
  C the Southern Irish
  D the Hutterites
  E northern Swedes

43 The 'drift' hypothesis
  A was supported by Goldberg and Morrison's findings (1963)
  B is consistent with the finding of high first admission rates for schizophrenia in the central zones of large cities
  C suggests that vulnerable individuals in poor, inner city areas drift into schizophrenia
  D was postulated by Faris and Dunham (1939) to explain their findings
  E is supported by the finding that schizophrenics were in similar status occupations to their fathers

42 A B C E

Böök (1953) reported a high prevalence rate of schizophrenia in a community in northern Sweden. He suggested a schizoid personality might assist survival in an isolated area.

There appear to be high prevalence rates also in the Tamils of southern India and Ceylon, the Southern Irish, the north-west Croatians and the Roman Catholic Canadians (Murphy, 1968).

Eaton and Weil (1955) reported an unusually low prevalence of schizophrenia in an anabaptist sect in North America called the Hutterites. However, Murphy (1968) was unable to confirm this.

Odegaard (1932) found schizophrenia was more prevalent in Norwegians who emigrated to America than in those who stayed behind.

Böök J.A. (1953) A genetic and neuropsychiatric investigation of a north-Swedish population. *Acta Genet. Stat. Med.* **4**, 1–15.
Eaton J.W. & Weil R.J. (1955) *Culture and Mental Disorders*. Glencoe, Illinois, The Free Press.
Murphy H.B.M. (1968) Cultural factors in the genesis of schizophrenia. In Rosenthal D. & Kety S. (eds) *The Transmission of Schizophrenia*. Oxford, Pergamon Press.
Odegaard O. (1932) Emigration and insanity. *Acta Psychiat.* Suppl. 4.

43 A B

Unusually high first admission rates for schizophrenia were reported by Faris and Dunham (1939) in the inner districts of Chicago. Similarly high rates have been found for other large cities.

Faris and Dunham put forward a *'breeder'* or *'social causation'* hypothesis, that the poverty and social disorganization of inner urban areas gave rise to schizophrenia in predisposed individuals.

However, findings of Goldberg and Morrison (1963) that schizophrenic patients were in lower status occupations than their fathers suggested that the patients had drifted down the social scale as a consequence of their illness-related handicaps—the *drift hypothesis*. A variant of this which implies a more active mechanism is the *'segregation' hypothesis*. This suggests that the pre-schizophrenic or schizophrenic individual gravitates to inner city areas in seeking out the anonymity they provide.

Faris R.E.L. & Dunham H.W. (1939) *Mental Disorders in Urban Areas. An Ecological Study of Schizophrenia and Other Psychoses*. Chicago, University of Chicago Press.
Goldberg E.M. & Morrison S.L. (1963) Schizophrenia and social class. *Br. J. Psychiat.* **109**, 785.

44 The morbid risk or lifetime expectancy of developing schizophrenia is
A   40 per cent if one parent is affected
B   10 per cent in the brother of a schizophrenic
C   70 per cent when both parents have schizophrenia
D   10 per cent if a grandparent is affected
E   3 per cent in the niece of someone with schizophrenia

44 B E

There is fairly good agreement among studies using European diagnostic criteria that the morbid risk of schizophrenia in children with both parents affected is about 40 per cent, in first degree relatives is about 10 per cent and in second degree relatives about 3 per cent (see also Question 32).

Shields J. (1978) Genetics. In Wing J.K. (ed.) *Schizophrenia. Towards a New Synthesis.* London, Academic Press.

Further reading

Bebbington P. & Kuipers E. (1982) Social management of schizophrenia. *Br. J. Hosp. Med.* **28,** 396–403.
Crow T.J., Johnstone E.C. & Owen F. (1979) Research on schizophrenia. In Granville-Grossman K. (ed.) *Recent Advances in Clinical Psychiatry—3.* Edinburgh, Churchill Livingstone.
Hirsch S.R. (1978) Current status of the parental causation hypothesis in schizophrenia. In Gaind R.N. & Hudson B.L. *Current Themes in Psychiatry 1.* London, The Macmillan Press.
Hirsch S.R. (1983) Psychosocial factors in the cause and prevention of relapse in schizophrenia. *Br. Med. J.* **286,** 1600–1.
Wing J.K. (1978) *Schizophrenia. Towards a New Synthesis.* London, Academic Press.
Wing J.K. & Wing L. (eds) (1982) *Psychoses of Uncertain Aetiology. Handbook of Psychiatry.* Vol. 3. Cambridge, Cambridge University Press.

Affective Disorders

45 **Morbidity risk in relatives of those with affective disorders is**
   A   higher if they are male as opposed to female
   B   for both bipolar and unipolar disorder if the proband has bipolar illnesss
   C   about 10 per cent if they are first degree relatives
   D   lower if they are related to bipolar rather than unipolar probands
   E   higher if the proband became ill at a younger age

46 **The following lend support to a monoamine hypothesis of affective disorder:**
   A   monoamine oxidase inhibitors (MAOIs) increase amine concentrations in central synapses
   B   depression may complicate L-dopa treatment of Parkinsonism
   C   reserpine may precipitate depression
   D   L-tryptophan may benefit depressed subjects
   E   amphetamines induce euphoria

45 B C E

The morbidity risk for first degree relatives of those with affective disorder is about 10–15 per cent. The risk is greater in female than in male relatives and also in relatives of those who became ill at a younger age.

Perris (1966) suggested that bipolar and unipolar affective disorders tend to breed true, i.e. unipolar illness is rare in the relatives of bipolar probands and vice versa. However, in other studies the separation is less clear and generally while relatives of unipolar probands have an increased risk of only unipolar illness, relatives of bipolar probands appear to be at risk of both bipolar and unipolar disorders.

Generally morbidity risks are higher for relatives of bipolar rather than unipolar probands.

Perris C. (1966) A study of bipolar manic depressive and unipolar depressive psychosis. *Acta Psychiat. Scand.* **42**, Suppl. 194.
Reveley A. & Murray R.M. (1980) The genetic contribution to the functional psychoses. *Br. J. Hosp. Med.* **24**, 166–71.

46 A C D E

The monoamine hypothesis of affective disorder in its original form postulated a deficiency of central monoamines in depression and an excess in mania. It was based on the depressant activity of reserpine, the antidepressant effects of tricyclic drugs and MAOIs and the euphoriant effect of amphetamines, given the actions of these drugs on central amine transmitter systems (see Questions 171, 182).

The original hypothesis is *not* supported by findings that L-dopa (a precursor of dopamine) may precipitate depression when given as treatment for Parkinsonism (Mindham et al., 1976) but is supported by evidence that L-tryptophan (a precursor of 5-hydroxytryptamine) may supplement the antidepressant action of MAOIs (Coppen et al., 1963). The status of L-tryptophan as an antidepressant when given alone is less clear.

Coppen A., Shaw D.M. & Farrell J.P. (1963) Potentiation of the antidepressant effect of monoamine oxidase inhibitors by tryptophan. *Lancet* I, 79–81.
Mindham R.H.S., Marsden C.D. & Parkes J.D. (1976) Psychiatric symptoms during L-dopa therapy for Parkinson's disease and their relationship to physical disability. *Psychol. Med.* **6**, 23–33.

47 Characteristic features of psychotic (endogenous) depression include
  A weight loss
  B initial insomnia
  C agitation
  D depressed mood unresponsive to circumstances
  E *déjà vu* experiences

48 The following are recognized aetiological theories of the premenstrual syndrome:
  A deficiency of oestrogen
  B pyridoxine excess
  C fluid retention
  D prolactin excess
  E deficiency of progesterone

47 A C D

In British and European psychiatry the terms *psychotic* and *endogenous* have usually been applied synonymously to a depressive syndrome characterized by diurnal variation of mood, early morning waking, weight loss, guilt and movement disturbance such as agitation or retardation. *Neurotic* or *reactive* has implied a syndrome of fluctuating depression, self-pity rather than guilt and perhaps initial insomnia, often accompanied by anxiety.

In North America, however, the term *psychotic* has been reserved for depressive illness which has included 'psychotic' features such as delusions or hallucinations, and the terms *reactive* and *endogenous* have meant more literally the presence or the absence of precipitating events. Hence, according to this system a neurotic depression need not necessarily be reactive and a psychotic depression may have discernable precipitants. This would accord with research findings (Brown and Harris, 1978) which suggest that patients with the 'endogenous' type of depression described above are as likely as those with the 'reactive' syndrome to have experienced severely threatening life events in the preceding months.

Brown G.W. & Harris T.O. (1978) *Social Origins of Depression: A Study of Psychiatric Disorder in Women*. London, Tavistock Publications.

48 C D E

There have been suggestions at various times that the premenstrual syndrome is caused by: an excess of oestrogen, an idiosyncratic sensitivity to oestrogen, a deficiency of progesterone or withdrawal reactions to either oestrogen or progesterone. Evidence is inconclusive. A reported link between predominantly oestrogenic oral contraceptives and symptoms such as depression, decreased libido and nausea lends support to the postulated role of oestrogen excess; however, women taking oral contraceptives appear, if anything, to complain less often of premenstrual problems (RCGP, 1974).

Premenstrual feelings of bloatedness, weight gain and mood disturbances have been related to fluid retention and specifically an activation of the serum-angiotensin-aldosterone system; however, the evidence is inconsistent.

There is little evidence, also, to support suggestions that premenstrual symptoms are due to either elevated prolactin levels or pyridoxine deficiency.

Royal College of General Practitioners (1974) *Oral Contraceptives and Health*. London, Pitman Medical.

Affective Disorders: Questions

49 The following characterize atypical (complicated) grief:
 A hypochondriacal symptoms similar to those suffered by the deceased during his last illness
 B searching behaviour
 C male sex
 D pseudohallucinations of the dead person
 E hostility towards people connected with the death such as doctors or clergy

50 Puerperal psychosis
 A usually presents within 48 hours of parturition
 B has a risk of recurrence in a subsequent pregnancy of between 10 and 20 per cent
 C is more likely where there is a family history of affective disorder
 D has a worse prognosis when affective rather than schizophrenia symptoms are dominant
 E has an incidence of 1 in 500 births, taking onset of within six months of parturition

49 A E

Patients with *atypical* or *complicated* grief as described by Wretmark (1959) and Parkes (1965) differ in certain respects from the typically grief-stricken. Most are women (93 per cent of Wretmark's and 81 per cent of Parkes' cases). Delayed reactions are more common, the duration of the disturbance tends to be longer and the intensity of the reaction more severe. The following are also more common: difficulty in accepting the loss sometimes to the extent of denial, feelings of guilt and self-blame, marked hostility towards individuals associated with the death and hypochondriacal symptoms mimicking symptoms suffered by the deceased during his last illness.

Manifestations of *normal* grief may include perceptual disturbances such as illusions, misidentifications, pseudohallucinations and a sense of the 'presence' of the deceased, searching behaviour such as returning to places previously visited with the deceased and clinging to the deceased's possessions (in its extreme form, 'mummification' i.e. retaining parts of the house in the exact condition in which the deceased left them).

Granville-Grossman K. (1971) Grief. In *Recent Advances Clinical Psychiatry.* pp. 180–90. Edinburgh, Churchill Livingstone.
Parkes C.M. (1965) Bereavement and mental illness. *Br. J. Med. Psychol.* **38,** 1–26.
Wretmark G. (1959) A study in grief reactions. *Acta Psychiat. Scand.* Suppl. 136. pp. 292–9.

50 B C E

Onset of puerperal psychosis is uncommon within the first 48 hours, but the condition starts within one week of delivery in 40 per cent of cases. Most of the remaining cases start during the next three months.

The International Classification of Diseases suggests that functional psychotic illnesses beginning after parturition should be classified as schizophrenia, depressive psychosis or manic psychosis according to the main clinical features. However, the clinical picture may be mixed and difficult to categorize in this way. When schizophrenic symptoms are dominant a worse prognosis is indicated.

51 Depressive illness may present as
 A shop-lifting
 B dementia
 C schizophrenia
 D Gilles de la Tourette syndrome
 E hypochondriasis

52 Recognized treatments for the premenstrual syndrome are
 A bromocriptine
 B oral progesterone
 C ECT
 D amphetamines
 E dydrogesterone

51 A B E

Depressed patients, particularly elderly ones, may be mistakenly considered demented because of poor performance on cognitive tests. This pseudodementia is, however, due principally to the depressive's defective attention and concentration.

In many instances of hypochondriasis the condition is primarily affective. Hypochondriacal delusions occur particularly in elderly depressed patients (involutional melancholia) and may be nihilistic as in Cotard's syndrome.

Particularly in a middle-aged women, shop-lifting may be a feature of a depressive illness.

Depression may also present as alcoholism, an anxiety state, sexual offences in middle-aged men, pain and hysterical conversion.

Arie T. (1983) Pseudodementia. *Br. Med. J.* **286**, 1301–2.
Carney M. (1983) Pseudodementia. *Br. J. Hosp. Med.* **29**, 312–18.
Gibbens T.C.N., Palmer C. & Prince J. (1971) Mental health aspects of shop-lifting. *Br. Med. J.* **III**, 612–15.
Kenyon F.E. (1976) Hypochondriacal states. *Br. J. Psychiat.* **129**, 1–14.

52 A E

The natural hormone, progesterone, is inactive when taken by mouth but has been administered for premenstrual symptoms either in the form of rectal or vaginal suppositories or as daily injections. However, several synthetic progestogens such as dydrogesterone (Duphaston) are available as oral preparations and are reportedly as effective as progesterone.

Oral contraceptives, particularly low-dose combination ones such as 'Microgynon 30' or progestogen-only preparations such as 'Micronor', may also be tried.

Bromocriptine which suppresses prolactin secretion is also used but side-effects such as postural hypotension and nausea may be a problem.

The postulated role of fluid retention has led to the use of diuretics. Spironolactone which is an aldosterone antagonist might be expected to have special advantages.

Psychoactive drugs such as minor tranquillizers, antidepressants or lithium may have a role in therapy but amphetamines or ECT are not indicated. Pyridoxine is relatively innocuous but of uncertain efficacy.

53 The following are characteristic features of mania:
A elation
B hypersomnia
C pressured speech
D 'made' acts
E social withdrawal

53 A C

Mania is characterized by elation, pressure of speech, physical overactivity, grandiosity and expansiveness.

It has been claimed that first rank symptoms of schizophrenia (e.g. 'made' acts) occur in a minority of patients (Taylor and Abrams, 1973) but are certainly not characteristic of mania.

Taylor M.A.T. & Abrams R. (1973) The phenomenology of mania. *Arch. Gen. Psychiat.* **29**, 520–2.

54 Match each of the following classifications of depression (A–E) with the name associated with it (1–5):
  A depressive spectrum disease and pure depressive disease
  B primary and secondary
  C hierarchical
  D unipolar and bipolar
  E type S and type J

  1 Pollitt
  2 Winokur
  3 Perris
  4 Feighner
  5 Foulds

55 Neurotic (reactive) depression is characterized by
  A nihilistic delusions
  B retardation
  C fluctuating depression of mood
  D hallucinatory voices
  E diurnal variation in mood

54 A2 B4 C5 D3 E1

In practice the diagnosis of 'neurotic' depression is arrived at by the exclusion of 'psychotic' depression. Foulds drew attention to this *hierarchical* scheme of diagnosis and has postulated a hierarchy model of classification for depression and other psychiatric disorder (Foulds and Bedford, 1975). Leonhard first categorized manic-depressive psychosis as *bipolar* or *unipolar* (he actually used the term 'monopolar') and this system has been developed by Angst and by Perris (1966). 'Bipolar' implied attacks of both manic and depressive psychosis and 'unipolar', recurrent depression or recurrent mania. Now, as unipolar mania is rare and following further family studies, recurrent mania is usually regarded as bipolar illness in which an episode of depression has not yet occurred.

The St Louis classification distinguishes between *primary* and *secondary* depression. The former occurs where there is no previous psychiatric history other than mania or depressive illness, while secondary depressive disorder follows another psychiatric illness or is accompanied by an incapacitating or life-threatening physical illness (Feighner *et al.*, 1972).

Winokur (1973) has subdivided unipolar depressive disorder into *depressive spectrum disorder* and *pure depressive disease*. The former affects typically young females with depressed female relatives and sociopathic or alcoholic male relatives, while pure depressive disease characteristically affects older men, and male and female relatives have an equal risk of depression.

Pollitt (1965) divided depression into *type S* and *type J*. In the former, disturbed physiology gives rise to a 'depressive functional shift' and somatic symptoms. Type J is justifiable or understandable in terms of the patient's circumstances, and physiological changes are absent.

Feighner J.P., Robins E., Guze S.B., Woodruff R.A., Winokur G & Munoz R. (1972) Diagnostic criteria for use in psychiatric research. *Arch. Gen. Psychiat.* **26,** 57–63.

Foulds G.A. & Bedford A. (1975) Hierarchy of classes of person illness. *Psychol. Med.* **5,** 181–92.

Kendell R.E. (1976) The classification of depressions: a review of contemporary confusion. *Br. J. Psychiat.* **129,** 15–28.

Perris C. (1966) A survey of bipolar and unipolar recurrent depressive psychoses. *Acta Psychiat. Scand.* Suppl. 194.

Pollitt J.D. (1965) Suggestions for a physiological classification of depression. *Br. J. Psychiat.* **11,** 489–95.

Winokur G. (1973) The types of affective disorders. *J. Nerv. Ment. Dis.* **156,** 82–96.

55 C

See Question 47.

Affective Disorders: Questions

56 Match each of the following classifications of depression (A–E) with the person (1–5) who described it:
- A 2 categories: endogenous, neurotic
- B 1 dimension: psychotic–neurotic continuum
- C 3 categories: anxious-tense, hostile, retarded
- D 2 dimensions: psychoticism, neuroticism
- E 4 categories: psychotic, anxious, hostile, young depressive with personality disorder

- 1 Overall
- 2 Eysenck
- 3 Roth
- 4 Paykel
- 5 Kendell

57 Maternity blues
- A is rare
- B occurs in or after the third week of the puerperium
- C is characterized by persistent depression
- D requires antidepressant medication
- E occurs in at least 50 per cent of women

56 A3 B5 C1 D2 E4

Studies by Roth and his colleagues in Newcastle using discriminant function analysis suggested that *endogenous* and *neurotic* depressions were distinct conditions (Carney *et al.*, 1965). Kendell failed to replicate these findings and suggested that a more appropriate concept was a *psychotic–neurotic* continuum (Kendell and Gourlay, 1970). A further dimensional model was postulated by Eysenck (1970); however, he considered that two dimensions of *psychoticism* and *neuroticism* were necessary to adequately account for the clinical variation in depression.

Using cluster analysis in studies of depressives Paykel (1971) arrived at four groups: *psychotic, anxious, hostile* and *young* depressives with personality disorder. Overall *et al.* (1966) using between-person factor analysis obtained three groups: *retarded, anxious* and *hostile* depressives.

Carney M.W.P., Roth M. & Garside R.F. (1965) The diagnosis of depressive syndromes and the production of ECT response. *Br. J. Psychiat.* **111**, 659–74.

Eysenck H.J. (1970) The classification of depressive illness. *Br. J. Psychiat.* **117**, 241–50.

Kendell R.E. & Gourlay J. (1970) The clinical distinction between psychotic and neurotic depression. *Br. J. Psychiat.* **117**, 257–60.

Overall J.E., Hollister L.E., Johnson M. & Pennington V. (1966) Nosology of depression and differential response to drugs. *JAMA* **195**, 946–64.

Paykel E.S. (1971) Classification of depressed patients: a cluster analysis derived grouping. *Br. J. Psychiat.* **118**, 275–88.

57 E

Maternity or *baby blues* affects more than 50 per cent of women in the first 10 days of the puerperium. The symptoms of weepiness, irritability, despondency and forgetfulness are usually mild and transient. Reassurance and emotional support are sufficient treatment.

The more severe *postnatal depression* occurs in or after the third week of the puerperium.

58 The following were found by Brown and Harris to increase the risk of depression, in the presence of a severely threatening life event or major difficulty:
A three or more children under the age of 14 living at home
B unemployment
C a schizoid personality
D loss of a father before the age of 11
E lack of a confiding relationship

58 A B E
Vulnerability factors contribute to depression only in the presence of a provoking agent. Brown and Harris (1978) found a woman was more at risk of depression if she lacked an intimate tie (a confiding relationship), had three or more children under the age of 14 at home, had lost her mother (but not her father) before the age of 11 or was unemployed. A severe life event or a major difficulty was a provoking factor.

Brown G.W. & Harris T. (1978) *Social Origins of Depression: A Study of Psychiatric Disorder in Women*. London, Tavistock Publications.

Further reading

Brandon S. (1982) Depression after childhood. *Br. Med. J.* **284,** 613–14.
Clare A.W. (1979) The treatment of premenstrual symptoms. *Br. J. Psychiat.* **135,** 576–9.
Clare A.W. (1982) *Psychiatric Problems in Women. Part 3: The Premenstrual Syndrome*. London, SK & F Publications.
Paykel E.S. & Copen A. (eds) (1979) *Psychopharmacology of Affective Disorders*. Oxford, Oxford University Press.
Paykel E.S. & Rowan P.R. (1979) Affective disorders. In Granville–Grossman K.L. (ed.) *Recent Advances in Clinical Psychiatry—3*. Edinburgh, Churchill Livingstone.
Paykel E.S. (ed.) (1982) *Handbook of Affective Disorders*. Edinburgh, Churchill Livingstone.
Snaith R.P. (1983) Pregnancy-related psychiatric disorder. *Br. J. Hosp. Med.* **29,** 450–6.
Wing J.K. & Wing L. (eds) (1982) *Psychoses of Uncertain Origin. Handbook of Psychiatry*. Vol 3. Cambridge, Cambridge University Press.

Suicide and Deliberate Self-Poisoning or Self-Injury

59 Suicide is more common in
   A the married
   B wartime
   C the winter
   D those who have made previous attempts
   E females

60 Match each of the following terms (A–D) with the person (1–4) who proposed it:
   A parasuicide
   B non-fatal deliberate self-harm
   C attempted suicide
   D deliberate self-poisoning or self-injury

   1 Stengel
   2 Morgan
   3 Kessel
   4 Kreitman

61 The following characterize subjects of parasuicide (or deliberate self-poisoning/injury):
   A upper social class
   B recent experience of adverse life events
   C male sex
   D about 1 per cent kill themselves in the year following an attempt
   E unemployment
   F young age

59 D

Suicide rates are high in the divorced, single and widowed. The married are at relatively low risk. Rates are higher in men than women and increase with age.

Suicide occurs more commonly in the spring and summer than in other seasons and between a third and a half of those who complete suicide have a history of previous attempts (Barraclough *et al.*, 1974; Kreitman, 1977).

Barraclough B., Bunch J., Nelson B. & Sainsbury P. (1974) A hundred cases of suicide: clinical aspects. *Brit. J. Psychiat.* **125,** 355–73.
Kreitman N. (1977) *Parasuicide.* London, John Wiley & Sons.

60 A4 B2 C1 D3

Following the separation into two groups, on clinical and epidemiological grounds, those who commit suicide and those who non-fatally harm themselves, inconsistencies in terminology have arisen when discussing the second group.

Stengel (1952) in using the term *attempted suicide* presupposed an intent of self-destruction. However, it is clear that many of these patients do not actually attempt to kill themselves and other terms have placed less emphasis on aetiology and intention. Hence the terms *deliberate self-injury and self-poisoning, non-fatal deliberate self-harm* and *parasuicide* proposed by Kessel (1965), Morgan *et al.* (1975) and Kreitman (1977) respectively. The first two of these terms are self-explanatory. Parasuicide refers to 'any act deliberately undertaken by a patient which mimics the act of suicide but which does not result in a fatal outcome'.

Kessel N. (1965) Self poisoning. *Br. Med. J.* **II,** 1265–70, 1336–40.
Kreitman N. (ed.) (1977) *Parasuicide.* London, John Wiley & Sons.
Morgan H.G., Pocock H. & Pottle S. (1975) The urban distribution of non-fatal deliberate self-harm. *Br. J. Psychiat.* **126,** 319–28.
Stengel E. (1952) Enquiries into attempted suicide. *Proc. R. Soc. Med.* **45,** 613–20.

61 B D E F

Generally parasuicide is more common in females, the divorced and single, the lower social classes and the unemployed. Most who deliberately poison or injure themselves are young—at least two-thirds are less than 35 years old, and the majority have recently experienced threatening or undesirable life events (Paykel *et al.*, 1975).

One to 2 per cent of parasuicide subjects kill themselves in the first year of follow-up (Kreitman, 1977).

Kreitman N. (ed.) (1977) *Parasuicide.* London, John Wiley & Sons.
Paykel E.S., Prusoff B.A. & Myers J.K. (1975) Suicide attempts and recent life events. *Arch. Gen. Psychiat.* **32,** 327–33.

62 Match each of the following kinds of suicide (A–D) as described by Durkheim with the appropriate social context (1–4):
    A egoistic
    B anomic
    C altruistic
    D fatalistic

    1 excessive integration
    2 poor integration
    3 excessive regulation
    4 poor regulation

62 A2 B4 C1 D3

Durkheim (1897) proposed a socially determined predisposition to suicide and considered that suicide was less common in well integrated and well regulated societies.

He suggested that where there is a sense of social isolation *egoistic* suicide occurs. In contrast where social integration is excessive and an individual kills himself for the 'general good', suicide is *altruistic*. *Anomic* suicide occurs typically in socially disorganized urban areas where there may be a discrepancy between an individual's aspirations and the values of society. Under conditions of excessive regulation, for instance in prison, fatalistic suicide may occur.

Durkheim E. (1897) *Le Suicide*. Translated in 1952 as *Suicide: A Study in Sociology* by Spaulding J.A. & Simpson G. London, Routledge & Kegan Paul.

63 **Available evidence suggests that**
   A   two-thirds of suicides have consulted their GP in the month before the act
   B   most cases of suicide are not mentally ill at the time
   C   alcoholism is the most common diagnosis in suicide patients
   D   only trained psychiatrists can safely assess parasuicide subjects
   E   suicide rates have decreased since 1961

63 A E

In a study of 100 suicides in West Sussex and Portsmouth, in which detailed histories were obtained from relatives and doctors soon after the subject had committed suicide, Barraclough et al. (1974) found that two-thirds of subjects had seen their GP in the month and 40 per cent in the week before the act. Psychiatric disorder was diagnosed in 94 per cent. This closely agrees with a corresponding finding of 93 per cent by Robins et al. (1959). In both studies the most frequent condition was depressive illness, with alcoholism second (the principal diagnosis in 70 per cent and 15 per cent respectively of cases in the Barraclough study).

The assessment of parasuicide subjects by staff other than psychiatrists has been evaluated. Findings suggest that house physicians (Gardner et al., 1977), social workers (Newson-Smith and Hirsch, 1979) and nurses (Catalan et al., 1980) are able to safely assess these patients.

Overall suicide rates have progressively fallen since 1961. The carbon monoxide content of domestic gas has been reduced since then and rates for suicide using this means have decreased. There appears to have been in general no compensatory increase in the use of other methods.

Barraclough B., Bunch J., Nelson B. & Sainsbury P. (1974) A hundred cases of suicide: Clinical aspects. *Br. J. Psychiat.* **125**, 355–73.
Catalan J., Marsack P., Hawton K.E., Whitwell D., Fagg J. & Bancroft J.H. (1980) Comparison of doctors and nurses in the assessment of deliberate self-poisoning patients. *Psychol. Med.* **10**, 483–91.
Gardner R., Hanka R., O'Brien V.C., Page A.J.F. & Rees R. (1977) Psychological and social evaluation in cases of deliberate self-poisoning admitted to a general hospital. *Br. Med. J.* **II**, 1567–70.
Newson-Smith J.G.B. & Hirsch S.R. (1979) A comparison of social workers and psychiatrists in evaluating parasuicide. *Br. J. Psychiat.* **134**, 335–42.
Robins E., Murphy G., Wilkinson R.H., Gassner S. & Kayes J. (1959) Some clinical considerations in the prevention of suicide based on a study of 134 successful suicides. *Am. J. Publ. Hlth.* **49**, 888–99.

Further reading

Suicide and parasuicide

Farmer R.D.T. & Hirsch S. (eds) (1980) *The Suicide Syndrome*. London, Croom Helm.
Hawton K. & Catalan J. (1981) Psychiatric management of attempted suicide patients. *Br. J. Hosp. Med.* **25**, 365–72.
Kreitman N. (1978) Social and clinical aspects of suicide and parasuicide (attempted suicide): a contribution from psychiatric epidemiology. In Forrest A., Affleck J. & Zealley A. (eds) *Companion to Psychiatric Studies*. pp. 30–43. Edinburgh, Churchill Livingstone.
Morgan H.G. (1982) Deliberate self-harm. In Granville-Grossman K. (ed.) *Recent Advances in Clinical Psychiatry—4*. pp. 47–74. Edinburgh, Churchill Livingstone.
Sainsbury P. (1981) Clinical aspectes of suicide and its prevention. In Crown S. (ed.) *Practical Psychiatry*. Vol. 1. pp. 50–4. London, Northwood Books.

Neurosis and Personality Disorder

64 **Hypochondriasis is**
 A more prevalent in lower social classes
 B more common in medical students
 C definable as a morbid preoccupation with one's body or state of health
 D usually secondary to some other disorder
 E less common in males

65 **The following statements relating to hysteria are true:**
 A female/male ratio in Briquet's syndrome is 3:2
 B Janet emphasized the importance of dissociation
 C an example of primary gain is gaining others' attention
 D Slater's study lent support to the concept of hysteria
 E amnesia is a conversion symptom

64 *A B C D*

Hypochondriasis appears to be usually part of another syndrome, most commonly a depressive illness. The status of primary hypochondriasis is controverisal.

Some groups are alleged to be particularly prone to hypochondriasis: the male sex, lower social classes, the very young, the old, Jews and medical students.

Kenyon F.E. (1964) Hypochondriasis: a clinical study. *Br. J. Psychiat.* **110**, 478–88.

65 *B*

Hysterical disorders may be *dissociative,* such as amnesic states and fugues, or *conversion states* in which bodily symptoms occur, according to psychoanalytic theory by the conversion of unconscious anxiety into a symptom of symbolic significance.

Janet emphasized, as a mechanism in hysteria, dissociation, i.e. a state of affairs whereby two or more mental processes coexist without becoming integrated.

Gain has been considered important to the concept of hysteria, *primary* gain being a relief from an intolerable intrapsychic conflict and *secondary* gain being the advantage which results from the disorder in terms of manipulating relationships or avoiding unwanted situations or tasks. Classically any gain in hysteria is unconscious and conscious motivation implies malingering, although it may be difficult to draw the distinction, which at any rate is often unhelpful when it comes to management.

In an influential study of 85 patients given a diagnosis of hysteria at the National Hospital, Queen Square, at follow-up nine years later, Slater found that in one-third of patients the diagnosis had been replaced by an organic one; 12 patients had died, 3 of diseases which could have accounted for the 'hysterical' symptoms; 13 had developed psychiatric illness. The findings were taken by many as evidence of weakness in the concept of hysteria.

Briquet's syndrome (St Louis hysteria) has not been described in males. The women described all had multiple symptomatology, unaccounted for by organic disease. Menstrual symptoms were particularly common. A familial bias for the syndrome has been claimed. The validity of the syndrome as a distinct diagnostic entity has been questioned.

Kendell R.E. (1974) A new look at hysteria. *Medicine,* 1st Ser, 1780–3.
Slater E. & Glithero E. (1965) A follow-up of patients diagnosed as suffering from hysteria. *J. Psychosom. Res,* **9,** 9–13.

Neurosis and Personality Disorder: Questions

66 Recognized features of anorexia nervosa include
A bradycardia
B hypercholesterolaemia
C hypertension
D distortion of body image
E erythema nodosum

67 For each numbered treatment of phobic anxiety select the lettered person or persons who described it:
A Frankl
B Jacobson
C Stampfl and Levis
D Wolpe
E Malleson

1 progressive relaxation
2 paradoxical intention
3 reactive inhibition therapy
4 systematic desensitization
5 implosion therapy

66 A B D

Bradycardia and *hypotension* occur secondary to starvation. Vomiters and purgers may, however, have a tachycardia.

Bruch regards distortion of body image as an essential feature of true anorexia nervosa, considering it 'a disturbance of delusional proportions'.

The causation of high serum cholesterol levels in anorexia nervosa is unclear. Crisp considers that they are related to the consumption of foods with a high cholesterol content such as cheese.

Erythema nodosum is not a recognized feature.

67 A2 B1 C5 D4 E3

Wolpe described a treatment method for phobias called *systematic desensitization*. This was based on a principle named *reciprocal inhibition*, which postulated that if a response incompatible with anxiety (such as relaxation) was produced, while the subject was exposed to the source of his anxiety, then the fear response would be extinguished.

The technique involves firstly establishing a hierarchy of fear provoking situations for the particular patient, who is then asked to imagine the increasingly difficult situations whilst relaxed. Relaxation may be produced by Jacobsen's method of *progressive relaxation*.

A radically different approach to treatment called *flooding* involves prolonged exposure to the feared object or situation. The prototypes of the modern technique of flooding were probably as follows:

1 *Paradoxical intention* introduced by Frankl—a treatment method which involved the patient paradoxically attempting to produce the symptoms.

2 A similar technique called *reactive inhibition therapy* and described by Malleson.

3 *Implosion therapy* described by Stampfl and Levis in which the patient was encouraged to imagine as vividly as possible a previously fearful situation with all its emotional connotations.

68 **In subjects with anorexia nervosa, at low weight, endocrine changes are as follows:**
  A elevated plasma cortisol levels
  B higher than normal thyroxine (T4) levels
  C lower than usual luteinizing hormone (LH) and follicular stimulating hormone (FSH) levels
  D abnormally high prolactin secretion
  E low growth hormone (GH) levels

68 A C

FSH and LH levels tend to be lower than usual in the circulation of anorexic subjects at low weight.

T4 levels are characteristically within the normal range although tending to be lower than those of matched controls. Thyroid stimulating hormone (TSH) levels are also near normal.

Prolactin levels are usually normal in subjects with anorexia nervosa. Dopamine antagonist drugs, such as chlorpromazine, tend to increase prolactin levels and may, therefore, complicate investigation.

Elevated levels of GH are usual in starving subjects. They revert to normal with refeeding.

An increased plasma cortisol level is usual. This is probably due to a reduction in the metabolic destruction of cortisol rather than to an increase in its production.

Neurosis and Personality Disorder: Questions

69 For each numbered concept select the lettered person who described it:
 A Miller
 B Parsons
 C Pilowsky
 D Asher
 E Mechanic

 1 Munchausen's syndrome
 2 illness behaviour
 3 accident neurosis
 4 sick role
 5 abnormal illness behaviour

69 *A3 B4 C5 D1 E2*

The concept of *illness behaviour* was proposed by Mechanic (1962) and refers to the ways in which symptoms are perceived, evaluated and acted upon by the individual. He has demonstrated how factors such as religion and social class influence how an individual acts in response to his symptoms, for instance his tendency to seek medical advice. Illness behaviour may be considered inappropriate given a person's situation and the degree of disability. This idea has been developed by Pilowsky (1969) as the concept of *abnormal illness behaviour*.

Parsons (1951) has described four features—actually two rights and two obligations of adopting the *sick role*: exemption from normal social responsibilities, not being held responsible for one's condition, an obligation to want to recover, and an obligation to seek the appropriate help agency, usually a doctor, and to cooperate with him.

Miller (1961) looked at cases with neurotic symptoms following head injury and chose the term *accident neurosis*. Although a number of patients grossly exaggerated their complaints, the conclusion was that true malingering was uncommon. Gross symptoms were inversely related to the severity of the head injury and seemed to occur most when the accident was perceived by the patient as someone else's fault and where financial compensation was a possibility.

Asher (1951) described *Munchausen's syndrome*. The typical patient feigns illness to bring about repeated hospital admissions and usually repeated investigations and operations. Barker (1962) has preferred the term 'hospital addiction syndrome'.

Asher R. (1951) Munchausen's syndrome. *Lancet* **I**, 339–41.
Barker J.C. (1962) The syndrome of hospital addiction (Munchausen syndrome). *J. Ment. Sci.* **108**, 167–82.
Mechanic D. (1962) The concept of illness behaviour. *J. Chron. Dis.* **15**, 189–94.
Miller H. (1961) Accident neurosis. *Br. Med. J.* **I**, 919–25.
Parson T. (1951) *'The Social System'*. The Free Press, Glencoe, Illinois.
Pilowsky I. (1969) Abnormal illness behaviour. *Br. J. Med. Psychol.* **42**, 347–51.

70 **The following statements accord with the Yerkes–Dodson law:**
A at a low level of anxiety further stimulation is associated with decreased performance
B the relationship between anxiety and performance is a straightforward one of negative correlation
C if an anxiety level is low, taking an anxiolytic drug may reduce performance
D anxiety and performance are unrelated
E a sudden drop in performance may result from stimulating further an already highly anxious subject

71 **Obsessional personality is associated with**
A schizophrenia
B Gilles de la Tourette syndrome
C depression
D obsessional neurosis
E anorexia nervosa

70 C E

The Yerkes–Dodson law describes how the relationship between anxiety and performance depends on the initial level of anxiety, shown as follows:

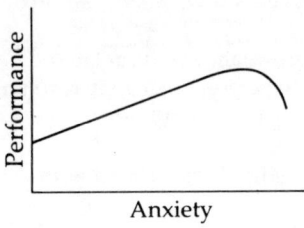

At a low level of anxiety performance increases with further stimulation. There is an optimal level of anxiety for performance, above which, however, performance suddenly deteriorates with a disruption of behaving patterns.

This law predicts that an anxiolytic would reduce performance in someone with low anxiety. Relief of anxiety, however, at the stage at which deterioration of performance occurs would not only relieve anxiety symptoms but also enhance performance.

71 C D E

Other associations of obsessional personality are with anxiety states, migraine and duodenal ulcer.

Associations of obsessional personality with schizophrenia or Gilles de la Tourette syndrome have not been recognized.

Black A. (1974) The natural history of obsessional neuroses. In Beech H.R. (ed.) *Obsessional States*. London, Methuen.

72 Characteristically, subjects with bulimia nervosa
A show signs of starvation
B do not regard the quantity of food eaten during a binge as excessive
C show *belle indifférence*
D are older than those with anorexia nervosa
E self-induce vomiting

73 Typically epidemic hysteria
A excludes minority groups
B occurs in males
C is instigated by an influential personality
D occurs in a setting of apprehension and concern
E happens in an institutional setting

72 D E

According to Russell's original diagnostic criteria (1979), subjects with bulimia nervosa (a) suffer from powerful and intractable urges to overeat, (b) seek to avoid the 'fattening' effects of food by inducing vomiting or abusing purgatives or both, and (c) have a morbid fear of becoming fat.

Nearly all such patients are female and, ranging in age from 16 to 40, are on average older than those with anorexia nervosa.

Characteristically, during a binge the quantity of food consumed is regarded as excessive and the eating is experienced as outside the subject's control. Between binges food intake is usually reduced. The patients are typically experts on dieting and may weigh themselves several times daily.

Depression, guilt feelings, suicidal ideation, anxiety and irritability are common; depression and guilt feelings are particularly pronounced immediately after a binge.

While metabolic complications of vomiting or purgative abuse such as dehydration, hypokalaemia and alkalosis may lead to cardiac arrhythmias, fits, tetany and peripheral paraesthesia, a balance between overeating and compensatory behaviour such as vomiting means that body weight is generally within the normal range and clinical signs of starvation are not present.

Russell G.F.M. (1979) Bulimia nervosa: an ominous variant of anorexia nervosa. *Psychol. Med.* **9,** 429.

73 A C D E

Epidemic hysteria refers to outbreaks of hysterical symptoms which have been described usually among young females, in institutions such as schools or convents. A background atmosphere of apprehension and tension is common and the behaviour is usually initiated by a powerful, influential individual, spreads to younger girls but excludes members of minority groups or outsiders such as very bright pupils.

Benaim S., Horder J. & Anderson J. (1973) Hysterical epidemic in a classroom. *Psychol. Med.* **3,** 366–73.

74 The following are true of phobias:
A the fear is proportional to the situation
B the provoking stimulus is avoided
C a fear of rats was induced in Albert
D agoraphobia is the type most commonly seen by psychiatrists
E the fear is under voluntary control

75 Match each of the following people (A–E) with the corresponding aetiological theory of anorexia nervosa (1–5):
A Russell
B Crisp
C Waller
D Lasègue
E Bruch

1 defence against unconscious fantasies of oral impregnation
2 'struggle for control, for a sense of identity and effectiveness'
3 weight phobia and an escape from the sexual demands of adolescence
4 disturbance of hypothalamic function
5 *anorexie hystérique*

74 B C D

A phobia may be defined as a fear which is disproportionate to the demands of the situation, is involuntary, cannot be reasoned away and leads to avoidance of the situation (Marks, 1969).

Watson described the induction of a fear of white rats in a child called Albert by repeatedly causing a loud noise behind him when he attempted to touch a white rat. Other experiments have demonstrated that fear responses can be produced by conditioning processes and provide evidence for phobias being learnt phenomena.

In 1909, Freud had described a phobia of horses in Little Hans, postulating that a fear of his father and specifically of castration was displaced on to horses.

Agoraphobia accounts for about 60 per cent of phobic patients seen by psychiatrists.

Marks I.M. (1969) *Fears and Phobias*. London, Heinemann Medical Books.

75 A4 B3 C1 D5 E2

Gull and Lasègue provided early descriptions of the condition. Gull named it 'anorexia nervosa' while Lasègue, involving the concept of hysteria, named it *anorexie hystérique*.

Psychoanalysts such as Waller have emphasized the role of fantasies of oral impregnation in aetiology.

Bruch has hypothesized that the 'relentless pursuit of thinness' of the anorexic subject represents a struggle for identity and effectiveness.

Crisp has suggested that the anorexic subject's avoidance of normal weight is a weight phobia and provides also a solution to adolescent turmoil in terms of avoidance of the demands, particularly sexual, of adolescence.

Russell (1977) has considered the evidence for a primary disturbance of hypothalamic function.

Gull W. (1873) Anorexia hysterica (apepsia hysterica). *Br. Med. J.* **II**, 527–8.
Lasègue C. (1983) De l'anorexie hystérique. *Archs. Gén. Méd.* **21**, 385–403.
Russell G.F.M. (1977) Editorial: the present status of anorexia nervosa. *Psychol. Med.* **7**, 363–7.
Waller J.V., Kaufman M.R. & Deutsch F. (1940) Anorexia nervosa. *Psychosom. Med.* **2**, 3–16.

76 **The following have been considered important in the aetiology of psychopathy:**
   A fixation at the anal stage of development
   B maternal deprivation in the first three years of life
   C 'double bind'
   D posterior temporal slow waves on the EEG
   E increased sensitivity of post-synaptic dopamine receptors

77 **The following statements concerning anxiety are true:**
   A a pill-rolling tremor is a sign
   B Freud related it to 'unconsummated sexual excitation'
   C the onset of trait anxiety can usually be defined
   D fear is a symptom
   E the patient may experience a sensation of choking

76 B D

Posterior temporal slow waves on the EEG have been found to be more common in psychopaths and this may reflect cerebral immaturity.

Bowlby regarded the period between the ages of nine months and three years as the time of maximal attachment behaviour, and proposed that maternal deprivation in the first three years of life could lead to psychopathy. A related viewpoint is that interference with early experience of bonding may result in later difficulties in social interaction.

Bateson hypothesized that the concept of 'double bind', whereby a child receives contradictory messages from a parent, was important in the aetiology of schizophrenia.

Freud related the development of the character traits of obstinacy, orderliness and parsimony to fixation at the anal stage of development (in the second year of life).

Tardive dyskinesia, a side-effect of long-term neuroleptic medication, may be due to hypersensitivity of dopamine receptors in the brain.

77 B D E

A useful distinction is between trait anxiety, which is a facet of personality, and state anxiety, which is a temporal disorder with a discernable time of onset.

Anxiety symptoms may be both psychological, such as fear and apprehension, and somatic, including palpitations, sweating, blushing, trembling, a dry mouth, dizziness, choking and smothering sensations.

An early theory of Freud was that anxiety represented repressed libido. A later theory that anxiety corresponded to a reliving of the birth experience was superseded by a theory that anxiety was a response of the ego to instinctual or emotional tension.

'Pill-rolling' describes the tremor in Parkinsonism.

Freud S. (1926) *Inhibitions, Symptoms and Anxiety*. Standard edition, Vol. 20. Hogarth Press, London, 1959.

Rycroft C. (1972) *A Critical Dictionary of Psychoanalysis*. Harmondsworth, Penguin Books.

78 **The following are recognized features of anorexia nervosa:**
   A carotenaemia
   B finger clubbing
   C lethargy
   D amenorrhoea
   E lanugo hair

78 A D E

Carotenaemia may be manifested as an orange-yellow pigmentation of the palms, soles and axillary folds. It is unlikely that an excessive intake of carotene-containing foods, such as carrots, entirely accounts for this.

Many regard amenorrhoea as an essential feature of anorexia nervosa. Reports vary on the timing of onset of the amenorrhoea and its relationship to weight loss. Crisp suggests that weight loss has occurred before amenorrhoea in almost all subjects and that nutritional changes are crucial to its causation. Russell, on the other hand, has reported patients in whom amenorrhoea appeared to precede other features. There is usually a delay of about nine months in the return of menses following restoration of normal weight.

Lanugo hair, secondary to starvation, grows on the back and limbs.

The anorexic subject is typically energetic and active. Finger clubbing is not a recognized feature.

Further reading

Bruch H. (1974) *Eating Disorders: Obesity, Anorexia Nervosa and the Person Within*. London, Routledge & Kegan Paul.
Crisp A.H. (1978) Anorexia nervosa. *Medicine, 3rd Ser.* **II**, 537–42.
Dally P., Gomez J. & Isaacs A.J. (1979) *Anorexia Nervosa*. London, Heinemann Medical Books.
Fairburn C.G. (1983) Bulimia nervosa. *Br. J. Hosp. Med.* **29**, 537–42.
Palmer R.L. (1982) Anorexia nervosa. In Granville-Grossman K. (ed.) *Recent Advances in Clinical Psychiatry—4*. pp. 101–22. Edinburgh, Churchill Livingstone.
Snaith P. *Clinical Neurosis*. Oxford, Oxford University Press.

Alcoholism

79 Postulated factors in the aetiology of alcoholism include
   A schism and skew
   B modelling
   C anal fixation
   D the finding that sons of alcoholics who are adopted, are no more likely than adoptees without alcoholic biological parents, to develop alcoholism
   E alcohol drinking to relieve anxiety

79 B E

Genetic factors do appear to be important in alcohol dependence. Goodwin *et al.* (1973) found that sons of Danish alcoholics who were adopted, were four times more likely than control adoptees to become alcoholic.

Psychoanalytical theories relate alcoholism to fixation at the *oral* (not anal) stage of development.

Alcoholism has been considered to be the consequence of vicarious learning (or modelling) from the drinking behaviour of parents or peers. Processes of classical or operant conditioning may also be important.

Alcohol may tranquillize the anxious or temporarily relieve the anguish of the depressed. A psychiatric condition underlying alcoholism should be looked for and treated if present.

Schism and skew are kinds of marital relationship considered by Lidz to be particularly prevalent in the parents of schizophrenics. These concepts have not been related to alcoholism.

Goodwin D.W., Schulsinger F., Hermansen L., Guze S.B. & Winokur G. (1973) Alcoholic problems in adoptees raised apart from alcoholic biological parents. *Arch. Gen. Psychiat.* **28,** 238–43.

80 **The following statements concerning the treatment of alcoholism are true:**
   A The efficacy of disulfiram implants is due to the high blood levels of disulfiram obtained
   B The Rand Report (Armor, Polich and Stambul, 1976) concluded that treatment produced no greater improvement than natural processes
   C Alanon is a self-help organization for family members of alcoholics
   D Controlled drinking should now be the aim of treatment for all patients
   E Orford and Edwards (1977) showed convincingly the efficacy of intensive treatment methods

80 C

The Rand Report gives the findings of a prospective study of 45 treatment centres for alcoholism in the USA. It was found that while 50 per cent of untreated patients had improved after 18 months, the corresponding figure for treated patients was 70 per cent. This greater improvement was not attributable to any particular treatment method. Patients who received only 'minimal' treatment, for instance one or two sessions after the initial assessment, showed a similar improvement rate to the untreated group. The conclusion was, 'the fact of treatment is more important than the specific type of treatment'; however, 'to produce a remission rate exceeding that due to natural processes, the treatment must be given in sufficient amounts'.

Edwards and colleagues carried out a study of 100 married, male alcoholics. Fifty received all available treatment facilities while the other half, matched on several variables, received only social worker follow-up after an initial assessment interview. At the end of one year the outcome in terms of drinking and social parameters was similar in the two groups. The authors suggested that treatment should be less intensive or interventionist.

Davies (1962) reported that seven of 93 alcoholics had returned to social drinking ten years after admission. Since then controlled or social drinking has been considered a possible outcome for certain patients. However, total abstinence should probably still be the aim of treatment when patients show signs of physical dependence.

With disulfiram implants, blood levels of disulfiram appear to be detectable, if at all, only in the first week after implantation. It appears that factors other than pharmacological deterrence are important with this form of treatment.

Self-help organizations in the area of alcoholism include Alcoholics Anonymous, Alanon (for family members and friends) and Al-Ateen (for teenage children of alcoholics).

Armor D.J., Polich J.M. & Stambul H.B. (1976) *Alcoholism and Treatment*. Santa Monica, Rand Corporation.
Davies D.L. (1962) Normal drinking in recovered alcohol addicts. *Q.L. Stud. Alcohol.* **23**, 94–104.
Orford J. & Edwards G. (1977) *Alcoholism*. Oxford, Oxford University Press.

81 10 grams of absolute alcohol are equivalent to
A 1 glass of sherry
B 2 glasses of wine
C 1 double measure of spirits
D 1 pint of beer
E 1 centilitre of absolute alcohol

82 Female alcoholics when compared to male alcoholics
A more often drink alone
B are more susceptible to liver cirrhosis
C commit fewer antisocial acts when intoxicated
D make more suicide attempts
E have a family history of alcoholism less often

83 Alcoholism is more common in
A Negroes than Whites in North America
B married than unmarried people
C Jews than non-Jews
D doctors than the general population
E the middle classes than other socio-economic classes

84 The Royal College of Psychiatrists recommends 'reasonable guidelines for the upper limit of drinking' per day of
A 4 single measures of spirits
B 1 standard-sized bottle of wine
C 60–80 g alcohol
D 8 glasses of sherry
E 4 pints of beer

81 A E

Standard measurement of quantity is required for valid epidemiological comparisons of alcoholism. Measurement of intake in grams of absolute alcohol per day is gradually being adopted for research and clinical purposes.

At present the standard unit in Britain is the centilitre, (approximately 10 g) of absolute alcohol, which is equivalent to half a pint of average-strength beer, a single measure of spirits, a glass of wine, or a small glass of sherry.

There are approximately 7 glasses to one standard-sized bottle of wine, 12 glasses to a bottle of sherry and 28 singles or tots to a bottle of spirits.

82 A B C D

Drinking problems among women appear to be on the increase. Women drinkers differ from their male counterparts in certain respects. They admit to greater appreciation of the psychological effects of alcohol and show less enjoyment of the drinking process itself. About 50 per cent drink alone. They have more alcohol-related problems and more often marital problems. The incidence of familial alcoholism is higher in female alcoholics.

83 A D

Alcoholism is more common in men than women. The age-group most affected is 40 to 54 years. It is least prevalent in the middle socio-economic classes and in the married. There is a relatively low prevalence in Jews. In North America the incidence is higher in Negroes than in Whites. Those involved in the manufacture, distribution and sale of alcohol are particularly at risk, along with company directors, commercial travellers, seamen, members of the armed forces, journalists, entertainers and doctors.

84 B C D E

The Royal College of Psychiatrists suggest than 'an intake of 4 pints of beer a day, 4 doubles of spirits or one standard-sized bottle of wine constitute reasonable guidelines for the upper limit of drinking' and state that it is 'unwise to make a habit of drinking even at these limits'. (One glass of sherry is roughly equivalent in alcohol content to 10 g absolute alcohol.)

These guidelines hold for men, but for women safe upper limits are considerably less, probably about half the amounts above.

Alcoholism: Questions

85 Recognized epidemiological indices of the prevalence of alcoholism include
 A per capita consumption of alcohol
 B hospital admissions with central pontine myelinolysis
 C divorce rates
 D mortality from liver cirrhosis
 E convictions for drunken driving

86 The following statements concerning alcoholism are true:
 A alcohol is mainly excreted unchanged
 B most people are clearly intoxicated with a blood alcohol level of 300 mg per cent
 C 'State dependent learning' refers to the need for sobriety when attempting to memorize material
 D acetaldehyde results from the action of alcohol dehydrogenase on alcohol
 E a blood alcohol level of 200 mg per cent is the British legal limit for driving

87 Alcohol drinking is associated with an increased incidence of
 A coronary artery disease
 B suicide
 C lung cancer
 D murder
 E tuberculosis

85 A D E

Indirect indices of the prevalence of alcoholism, used in epidemiological studies, include the per capita consumption of alcohol, mortality from liver cirrhosis, hospital admissions for alcoholism, convictions for drunken driving and convictions for drunkenness.

The distribution of drinkers to consumption is represented by a log-normal curve with a positive skew. This curve being continuous and unimodal suggests that social drinking and alcoholism are only quantitatively different in development, and that alcohol dependence is connected more with social properties such as the cost and availability of alcohol rather than individual predisposition.

The prevalence of alcoholism may be estimated from the mortality rate for liver cirrhosis using the Jellinek formula.

Central pontine myelinolysis is a rare complication of alcoholism and is unlikely to provide a useful index. Divorce is related to many different things and is likely to be too indirect an index to be of value.

86 B D

Up to 5 per cent of ingested alcohol is excreted unchanged in the kidneys and lungs. The rest is metabolized in the liver, by alcohol dehydrogenase, to acetaldehyde, which is in turn metabolized to acetate and ultimately to water and carbon dioxide.

A blood alcohol level of 80 mg per cent is the statutory limit for driving in Great Britain. At a level of 300 mg per cent the majority of people are obviously intoxicated; a level of more than 500 mg per cent may be fatal.

Material learned in a state of intoxication may be recalled better while in a similar state. This is an example of state dependent learning.

87 B C D E

The two most important psychiatric conditions in suicides are affective disorder and alcoholism. Between six and ten per cent of hospitalized alcoholics commit suicide (Kessel and Grossman, 1961).

The association with lung cancer may be due to more smoking in heavy drinkers. Tuberculosis in drinkers may be related to factors such as undernutrition, poor self-care and hygiene.

There is evidence that up to one half of murderers have been drinking before the act (Virkkunen, 1974).

Coronary artery disease is no more common in alcohol drinkers and moderate alcohol drinking may have a protective effect.

Kessel N. & Grossman G. (1961) Suicide in alcoholics. *Br. Med. J.* **II**, 1671–2.
Virkkunen M. (1974) Alcohol as a factor precipitating aggression and conflict behaviour leading to homicide. *Br. J. Addict.* **69**, 149–54.

88 Match each of Jellinek's types of alcoholism (A–E) with the appropriate clinical description (1–5):
A alpha
B beta
C gamma
D delta
E epsilon

1 drinking to relieve physical or psychological pain
2 loss of control drinking
3 bout drinking
4 inability to abstain from drinking
5 physical complications from a cultural pattern of drinking and poor nutrition

89 The following are features of the 'alcohol dependence syndrome' as described by Edwards and Gross (1976):
A altered tolerance to the effects of alcohol
B personality deterioration
C marital problems
D alcoholic hepatitis
E repeated withdrawal symptoms

90 The following are true of alcoholic withdrawal states:
A untreated delirium tremens has a mortality of 15 per cent
B chlordiazepoxide is a suitable sedative
C hypoglycaemia is a complication
D delirium tremens typically occurs 12 hours after cessation of drinking
E 'rum fits' occur in the first 48 hours

88 A1 B5 C2 D4 E3

Although Jellinek's classification may still be useful to clinicians, there is evidence that many drinkers do not adhere to any one pattern of alcoholism but show different types of drinking at different times.

Jellinek E.M. (1960) *The Disease Concept of Alcoholism.* New Jersey, Hillhouse Press.

89 A E

Features of the alcohol dependence syndrome are
1 Subjective awareness of a compulsion to drink
2 Narrowing of the drinking repertoire
3 Primacy of drinking over other activities
4 Altered tolerance to alcohol
5 Repeated withdrawal symptoms
6 Relief or avoidance of withdrawal symptoms by further drinking
7 Reinstatement after abstinence

Marital problems, personality deterioration and alcoholic hepatitis are examples of *alcohol-related disabilities*.

Edwards G. & Gross M.M. (1976) Alcohol dependence: provisional description of a clinical syndrome. *Br. Med. J.* **I**, 1058–61.

90 A B C E

The following withdrawal states may occur in the first 48 hours after stopping drinking:
1 A tremulous state consisting of tremor, nausea, vomiting and anxiety and sometimes called 'the shakes'.
2 An hallucinatory state in which hallucinations, usually visual, and other perceptual disturbances occur, known as 'the horrors'.
3 Grand mal seizures or 'rum fits'.

Delirium tremens usually occurs three to four days after cessation of drinking. It is a confusional state with clinical features of restlessness, disorientation, illusions, hallucinations, delusions and an affect of fear. Untreated it presents risks and has a mortality rate of about 15 per cent.

Complications of alcohol withdrawal include hypoglycaemia, hyponatraemia, hypokalaemia, hypomagnesaemia and respiratory alkalosis.

Chlordiazepoxide and chlormethiazole are suitable sedatives to use. A suitable starting dose of chlordiazepoxide is 20 to 30 mg 6-hourly, reducing gradually over five days, although higher doses may be required.

91 **In alcoholic hallucinosis**
   A the patient is confused
   B hallucinations are usually visual
   C some patients progress to schizophrenia
   D the cause is thiamin deficiency
   E auditory hallucinations are usually experienced as pleasant

92 **The following conditions are associated with the corresponding pathological or clinical features:**
   A Zieve's syndrome
   B 'fetal alcohol syndrome'
   C Marchiafava–Bignami disease
   D Mallory–Weiss syndrome
   E Korsakoff's psychosis

   1 lesions of the mammillary bodies
   2 laceration of the oesophagus
   3 haemolytic anaemia
   4 degeneration of the corpus callosum
   5 craniofacial abnormalities

93 **Recognized features of Korsakoff's psychosis include**
   A thiamin deficiency
   B a subsequent clinical picture of Wernicke's encephalopathy
   C retrograde amnesia
   D apathy
   E unimpaired new learning ability

91 C

Alcoholic hallucinosis is characterized by auditory hallucinations in clear consciousness. The 'voices' are usually unpleasant, for instance accusing the patient of sexual offences. It may occur at times of either relative decrease or increase in alcohol consumption. The causation and indeed the nature of the syndrome is unclear. There has been dispute over whether it is a type of organic brain disease, a form of schizophrenia or part of the alcohol withdrawal syndrome. On follow-up a minority of patients progress to schizophrenia.

92 A3 B5 C4 D2 E1

Pathological lesions in *Korsakoff's psychosis* are situated in the thalamic nuclei and the mammillary bodies. (See also Question 93.)

Mallory–Weiss syndrome refers to haematemesis caused by a tear at the lower end of the oesophagus. This commonly occurs after prolonged retching or vomiting, typically in alcoholics but also from causes such as migraine and pancreatitis.

There is increasing evidence that a mother's heavy drinking (at least a couple of bottles of wine each day or its equivalent) can damage the fetus and the *fetal alcohol syndrome* has been described in children of such mothers. Recognized features include low birth weight, mental retardation, an abnormally small head, congenital dislocation of the hips, congenital heart disease and cleft palate.

Zieve's syndrome is the association of haemolytic anaemia with cirrhosis, hyperlipidaemia and jaundice in alcoholics.

Marchiafava–Bignami disease is a rare alcohol-related condition characterized by degeneration of the corpus callosum.

Burton J.L. (1978) Harmful effects of alcohol. In Burton J.L. (ed.) *Aids to Postgraduate Medicine*, 3rd edn. pp. 93–4. Edinburgh, Churchill Livingstone.

Hore B.D., Heaton K.W., Bridgen W., Hanson J.W. & Pearce J.M.S. (1977) Alcoholism. *Br. J. Hosp. Med.* **18,** 106–43.

93 A C D

Wernicke's encephalopathy and Korsakoff's psychosis are successive syndromes (normally occurring in that order) of the same disease process which is due to thiamin deficiency.

Korsakoff's psychosis is characterized by a difficulty in learning new material, usually with a retrograde amnesia also, extending back for about one year prior to the onset of the psychosis, but sometimes longer. Other features found in some cases include confabulation, lack of insight, diminished drive and apathy.

94 Recognized features of Wernicke's encephalopathy include
A clear consciousness
B pathological changes to the mammillary bodies
C ocular muscle palsies
D vitamin B_6 deficiency
E nystagmus

94 B C E

Wernicke's encephalopathy is caused by deficiency of vitamin B_1 (thiamin), not vitamin B_6 (pyridoxine). Although usually associated with alcoholism it may arise from other causes of vitamin B_1 deficiency such as inadequate diet and *hyperemesis gravidarum*.

It is characterized by confusion, nystagmus, ocular palsies and ataxia, and is usually accompanied by polyneuropathy.

Further reading

Alcohol problems. ABC of alcohol. Alcohol and alcoholism. In *Articles from the British Medical Journal*. (1982) London, British Medical Journal.
Cutting J. (1979) Alcohol dependence and alcohol-related disabilities. In Granville-Grossman K. (ed.) *Recent Advances in Clinical Psychiatry—3*. pp. 225-50. Edinburgh, Churchill Livingstone.
Cutting J. (1982) Alcoholism: neuropsychiatric complications of alcoholism. *Br. J. Hosp. Med.* **27**, 335-42.
Edwards G. (1982) *The Treatment of Drinking Problems. A Guide for the Helping Professions*. London, Grant McIntyre.
Hore B.D. (1976) *Alcohol Dependence*. London, Butterworth.
Murray R. (1979) Alcoholism. In Hill P., Murray R. & Thorley A. (eds) *Essentials of Postgraduate Psychiatry*. pp. 319-48. London, Academic Press.
Murray R.M. & Gurling H.M.D. (1982) Alcoholism: polygenic influence on a multifactorial disorder. *Br. J. Hosp. Med.* **27**, 328-34.
Royal College of Psychiatrists (1979) *Alcohol and Alcoholism, Report of a Special Committee*. London, Tavistock Publications.

Drug Dependence

95 Recognized effects of amphetamines include
   A   bradycardia
   B   increased capacity for concentration
   C   meiosis
   D   tremor
   E   goose flesh

96 The following are true of cannabis:
   A   it lowers intra-ocular pressure
   B   it is extracted from the hemp plant
   C   physical dependence occurs in about 30 per cent of users
   D   dihydrocannibol is the main active ingredient
   E   marijuana is formed from the resin of the plant

97 Recognized complications of heroin addiction include
   A   nephrotic syndrome
   B   serum hepatitis
   C   cardiomyopathy
   D   optic neuritis
   E   carcinoma of the bronchus

95 B D

Early effects of amphetamines are euphoria, increased energy, restlessness, heightened powers of concentration and reduced hunger. Later *tachycardia*, increased reflexes and dilated pupils (mydriasis not meiosis) occur; and later still ataxia, tremor and slurring of speech.

'Goose flesh' is a feature of heroin withdrawal.

96 A B

Cannabis is derived from the hemp plant *(Cannabis sativa)*. The two main forms are *marijuana*, from the dried flowering tops and leaves, and hashish, a resinous extract. *Tetra*hydrocannibol is the main active substance.

Cannabis is either smoked or ingested in food or drinks. While physical dependence does not seem to occur, some users develop psychological dependence.

Psychological effects of taking the drug include feelings of contentment and relaxation, and perceptual distortions. Perception of time may be disturbed so that experiences lasting only seconds may seem to occupy hours or days. Flashback experiences sometimes occur.

Physical effects include tachycardia, conjunctival injection and lowered intra-ocular pressure. Gynaecomastia is an uncommon sequela. Other reported but less well-substantiated sequelae of cannabis use are acute or chronic psychotic illness, the 'amotivational syndrome', decreased spermatogenesis, brain damage with dilated cerebral ventricles and teratogenic effects.

97 A B

Complications include thrombophlebitis, gangrene, serum hepatitis, tuberculosis, endocarditis, nephrotic syndrome and transverse myelitis.

Cardiomyopathy and optic neuritis are complications of alcoholism and bronchial carcinoma complicates tobacco smoking.

98 The following statements concerning cocaine are true:
A 'snorting' causes nasal ulceration
B its effects were described by Sigmund Freud
C visual hallucinations are characteristic of cocaine-induced psychosis
D it is a derivative of coca
E according to the Misuse of Drugs Act 1971, it is a Class B drug

99 Indications for the prescription of amphetamines include
A narcolepsy
B obesity
C anorexia nervosa
D depressive illness
E hyperkinetic syndrome

100 Stimson (1973) divided heroin addicts into the following types:
A 'two-worlders'
B 'stables'
C 'loners'
D 'mainliners'
E 'drop-outs'

98 *A B D*

Cocaine, which was derived from coca, is a Class A drug. It may be sniffed ('snorted'), chewed or injected intravenously. Ulceration of the nasal mucosa is a complication of sniffing.

A paranoid psychosis, similar to that induced by amphetamines, can follow use of cocaine, especially chronic high dosage. Tactile hallucinations are characteristic, particularly hallucinations of crawling insects (formication)—hence the so-called 'cocaine bug'.

Freud studied the effects of cocaine by self-administration and by giving it in experiments to colleagues and patients. His paper *Uber Coca* published in July 1884 described its stimulant properties, and alluded to its anaesthetizing effects, although these were subsequently elucidated in more detail by Koller.

Clarke R.W. (1982) *Freud, The Man and The Cause.* pp. 59–62. London, Granada.

99 *A E*

Amphetamines have been prescribed for depression and obesity, particularly in the 1940s and 1950s. However, in view of the considerable potential for psychological dependence and possibly also physical dependence with this class of drugs, and because more effective drugs are now available at least for depressive illness, these conditions are not now indications for the use of amphetamines.

Amphetamines might be expected to aggravate some of the features of anorexia nervosa in view of their propensity to reduce appetite and increase activity.

Recognized indications for the prescription of amphetamines include narcolepsy and hyperkinetic syndrome (see Question 129).

100 *A B C*

Stimson described:
1 'Stables' who were generally law-abiding, employed and not involved in the drug scene.
2 'Loners' who tended to drift around, without much involvement in the drug culture or crime.
3 'Junkies' who were typically unemployed, involved in the drug scene and often in related crime such as 'pushing' drugs.
4 'Two-worlders' who combined characteristics of 'stables' and 'junkies' in that while they maintained a job and showed few complications of drug addiction they also participated in the drug culture and criminal activities.

Stimson G.V. (1973) *Heroin and Behaviour: Diversity Among Addicts Attending London Clinics.* Shannon, Irish University Press.

Drug Dependence: Questions

101 The following statements are true of heroin addiction:
 A physical dependence occurs only if the intravenous route of administration is adopted
 B according to the Misuse of Drugs Act 1971 heroin is a Class C drug
 C heroin was first used clinically as treatment for morphine addiction
 D under the 1973 Notification of and Supply to Addicts Regulations heroin addicts should be notified to the Royal College of Psychiatrists
 E any doctor who is fully registered is authorized to prescribe heroin in the treatment of addiction

102 Recognized features of withdrawal from barbiturates are
 A rhinorrhoea
 B tremor
 C grand mal seizures
 D increase in amount of rapid eye movement (REM) sleep
 E hypersomnia

103 Recognized clinical features of heroin withdrawal include
 A yawning
 B constipation
 C meiosis
 D lacrimation
 E goose flesh

101 C

The Misuse of Drugs Act 1971 placed drugs into three classes. Heroin is in Class A along with opium, morphine, methadone, pethidine, LSD, mescaline, psilocybin, cocaine and cannabinol. In Class B are amphetamine, d-amphetamine and cannabis, and in Class C benzphetamine and methaqualone.

Under the Misuse of Drugs Regulations 1973 (Notification of and Supply to Addicts) addicts to certain drugs including heroin should be notified by doctors to the Chief Medical Officer at the Home Office. Also only doctors with a Home Office Licence are authorized to prescribe heroin, morphine or cocaine in the treatment of addiction.

Heroin may be taken by mouth, by injection—intravenous, intramuscular or subcutaneous, by smoking it in a cigarette or by burning it otherwise and inhaling the fumes.

Physical dependence can occur whichever route is adopted.

102 B C D

Withdrawal symptoms include tremor, confusion, perceptual disturbances, grand mal seizures, anxiety and *insomnia* (not hypersomnia) with a rebound in the amount of REM sleep and dreaming.

Rhinorrhoea occurs in withdrawal from heroin.

103 A D E

Recognized features are rhinorrhoea, yawning, sweating, lacrimation, 'goose flesh', nausea, vomiting, abdominal cramps, diarrhoea (not constipation) and *mydriasis* (as a rebound from the meiosis of taking heroin).

Further reading

Edwards G. & Hawks S. (1973) *Terminology and Criteria of Drug Dependence.* Copenhagen, WHO.
Granville-Grossman K.L. (1979) Psychiatric aspects of cannabis use. In Granville-Grossman K.L. (ed.) *Recent Advances in Clinical Psychiatry—3.* pp. 251–70. Edinburgh, Churchill Livingstone.
Madden J.S. (1979) *A Guide to Alcohol and Drug Dependence.* Bristol, John Wright & Sons.
Murray R.M. (1981) Analgesic abuse. In Crown S. (ed.) *Practical Psychiatry.* Vol. 1. pp. 164–7. London, Northwood Books.
Thorley A. (1979) Drug dependence. In Hill P., Murray R. & Thorley A. (eds) *Essentials of Postgraduate Psychiatry.* pp. 277–318. London, Academic Press.

Sexual Dysfunction

104 Masters and Johnson described the following phases of sexual response:
A regression
B empathy
C resolution
D spontaneity
E excitement

105 The following are associated with good outcome in the treatment of sexual dysfunction:
A vaginismus
B alexithymia
C low sex drive
D non-sexual psychopathology
E premature ejaculation

106 According to Kinsey *et al.*
A 75 per cent of men experienced orgasm within two minutes of penetration
B about 40 per cent of men experienced homosexual orgasm by the age of 45
C 75 per cent of women had achieved orgasm during the first year of marriage
D 6.7 per cent of men under the age of 20 had erectile impotence
E men have a peak of sexual activity in their early 30s

104 C E

Four phases were described by Masters and Johnson (1966): excitement, plateau, orgasm and resolution. During the excitement and plateau stages genital vasocongestion results in erection in the male, and swelling and lubrication in the female. Arousal is maintained during the plateau phase until orgasm occurs.

There are two components to male orgasm, emission during which contraction of the internal reproductive organs occurs, and ejaculation brought about by perineal muscle contraction. Female orgasm is an ejaculatory equivalent, there is no stage corresponding to emission.

Masters W.H. & Johnson V.E. (1966) *Human Sexual Response*. Boston, Little, Brown & Company.

105 A E

Generally, sexual dysfunction has a good prognosis if it is of recent, acute onset in a couple with an otherwise good relationship, without other psychological difficulties and motivated to improve.

Of the specific problems treated by behavioural methods vaginismus and premature ejaculation show the best results. Sexual dysfunction arising from low sex drive is particularly difficult to treat. Also difficult to help are those people, often referred from non-psychiatric clinics, who tend to somatize their problems—consider them in physical terms only. Termed 'alexithymics' they include some with hypochondriacal neurosis, dysmorphophobia or monosymptomatic psychosis.

Crown S. & D'Ardenne P. (1982) Symposium on sexual dysfunction. Controversies, methods, results. *Br. J. Psychiat.* **140,** 70–7.

106 A B C

Kinsey and his colleagues (1948, 1953) provided extensive epidemiological data on human sexual behaviour.

They found the prevalence of erectile impotence increased from 0.1 per cent of men under 20, to 6.7 per cent of 40- to 50-year-old men to 75 per cent of men over 70.

Generally men peaked in sexual activity in late adolescence and women in their early 30s.

Kinsey A.C., Pomeroy W.B. & Martin C.E. (1948) *Sexual Behaviour in the Human Male*. Philadelphia, W.B. Saunders Company.
Kinsey A.C., Pomeroy W.B., Martin C.E. & Gebhard P.H. (1953) *Sexual Behaviour in the Human Female*. Philadelphia, W.B. Saunders Company.

107 Masters and Johnson treatment techniques for sexual dysfunction include:
 A stop-start technique
 B use of two therapists
 C daily treatment for two weeks
 D sensate focus
 E graded stimulation

107 B C D E

Masters and Johnson (1970) introduced a two-week residential treatment programme for sexual dysfunction (however, weekly treatment sessions with homework tasks have also proved successful). Each couple is treated by two therapists. Initially sexual attitudes are discussed and sexual information given. During the next stage of *sensate focus* mutual caressing progresses from non-sexual to sexual body areas with a ban imposed on intercourse. Later appropriate techniques are introduced for specific problems: graded stimulation (for erectile impotence or anorgasmia), graded dilators or finger exploration of the vagina (for vaginismus), superstimulation (for ejaculatory failure), and the squeeze technique described by Masters and Johnson, or alternatively the stop-start method (Kaplan, 1975), for premature ejaculation.

Kaplan H.S. (1975) *The New Sex Therapy*. London, Baillière Tindall.
Masters W.H. & Johnson V.E. (1970) *Human Sexual Inadequacy*. London, Churchill Livingstone.

Further reading

Bancroft J. (1979) Sex therapy. In Bloch S. (ed.) *An Introduction to the Psychotherapies*. pp. 146–71. Oxford, Oxford University Press.
Frank O.S. (1982) The therapy of sexual dysfunction. Br. J. Psychiat. **140**, 78–84.
Hawton K. (1982) The behavioural treatment of sexual dysfunction. Brit. J. Psychiat. **140**, 94–101.
Hawton K. (1982) Major common symptoms in psychiatry: sexual problems. Br. J. Hosp. Med. **27**, 129–35.

Organic Psychiatry

108 Clinical and pathological features of the punch-drunk syndrome include
   A   numerous senile plaques
   B   pyramidal signs
   C   increased tolerance of alcohol
   D   *cavum septi pellucidi*
   E   ataxia

109 The following are recognized features of delirium:
   A   impaired attention
   B   misidentifications
   C   nocturnal improvement
   D   formal thought disorder
   E   blunted affect

110 The following occur in dementia:
   A   impairment of consciousness
   B   perseveration
   C   dyscalculia
   D   catastrophic reactions
   E   amnesia for recent events

108 B C D E
Common early signs of *punch-drunkenness* or 'chronic traumatic encephalopathy of boxers' are ataxia and dysarthria, but varying combinations of cerebellar, extrapyramidal and pyramidal signs occur in the fully developed syndrome. Epilepsy often develops and intolerance of alcohol is characteristic. Psychiatric features include intellectual impairment, personality change often with irritability and outbursts of temper, and morbid jealousy.

Characteristic pathological changes are a widening of the space between the two leaves of the septum pellucidum *(cavum septi pellucidi)* and perforation or fenestration of the septum. Neurofibrillary tangles occur as in Alzheimer's disease, but senile plaques are virtually absent.

109 A B
Delirium implies a confusional state with also perceptual disturbances such as illusions or hallucinations.

The delirious patient has impaired attention or is distractible, and bizarre behaviour may follow from an incorrect grasp of his situation. Disorientation for time, place and person tends to develop in that sequence; misidentifications are common. Paranoid ideas may occur, sometimes delusional in quality, and mood is often one of fear although it may be labile. A fluctuating course and a worsening of symptoms at night are characteristic.

110 B C D E
Dementia is a global impairment of intellectual function, *in clear consciousness*, often associated with personality deterioration.

Amnesia for recent events tends to occur before memory is lost for remote events.

Perseveration, the continuation of a response after the appropriate stimulus has been withdrawn, is a recognized feature of dementia, as is the catastrophic response, an excessive emotional reaction to frustration.

Dementia need not be progressive or irreversible.

111 Match each of the following conditions (A–E) to the appropriate site of lesion (1–5):
A Gerstmann's syndrome
B constructional apraxia
C receptive dysphasia
D dysmnesic syndrome
E Broca's dysphasia

1 inferior frontal gyrus
2 superior temporal gyrus
3 angular gyrus
4 parietal lobe
5 hippocampus

112 The following statements concerning the EEG are true:
A 10–15 per cent of normal people have some abnormality on the EEG
B theta rhythm is 8–13 c/s
C 30 per cent of epileptics have normal interictal EEGs
D delta activity is normally only seen in very young children
E alpha rhythm disappears when the eyes are closed

111 A3 B4 C2 D5 E1

Bilateral medial temporal lobe damage, particularly bilateral *hippocampal* injury, is associated with a relatively pure dysmnesic syndrome. However, the dysmnesic syndrome as a result of chronic alcoholism (Korsakoff's psychosis) which is associated with confabulation, personality change and lack of insight is based on diencephalic damage.

Constructional apraxia (an ability to reproduce simple designs) occurs more often with right-sided than left-sided *parietal lobe* lesions but has been reported with bilateral damage.

Gerstmann's syndrome has been attributed to left-sided or dominant *angular gyrus* lesions (see also Question 114).

Broca's dysphasia (expressive or motor dysphasia) results from a lesion of the posterior part of the *inferior frontal gyrus*. Spoken words are slow and sparse. Comprehension is unaffected.

Wernicke's dysphasia (receptive or sensory dysphasia) occurs with posterior lesions of the *superior temporal gyrus*. Speech is paraphasic and fluent. Comprehension is impaired.

Nominal dysphasia is of little localizing value and occurs to some extent in all forms of dysphasia.

Lishman W.A. (1978) Symptoms and syndromes with regional affiliations. In *Organic Psychiatry*. pp. 29–108. Oxford, Blackwell Scientific Publications.

Robertson E.E. (1978) Organic disorder. In Forrest A.D., Affleck J.W. & Zealley A.K. (eds) *Companion to Psychiatric Studies*. pp. 459–98. Edinburgh, Churchill Livingstone.

Wilson L.A. (1980) Higher cerebral function. *Medicine, 3rd Ser.* **31**, 1621–3.

112 A C

Alpha rhythm is 8–13 c/s, beta more than 13 c/s, delta less than 4 c/s and theta 4–7 c/s.

Delta activity is seen normally not only in very young children but also during sleep.

Alpha rhythm is present when the person is fully awake but has his eyes closed. It attenuates when the eyes are opened or when mental activity such as mental arithmetic is carried out.

113 The following are usually associated with parietal lobe lesions of the non-dominant (subordinate) hemisphere:
   A neglect of the left half of visual space
   B *witzelsucht*
   C prosopagnosia
   D hemisomatognosia
   E ideomotor apraxia

114 **Gerstmann's syndrome consists of**
   A crossed laterality
   B dyscalculia
   C astereognosis
   D finger agnosia
   E dysphagia

113 A C D

Signs of non-dominant parietal lobe disease include neglecting the left side of the body (hemisomatognosia), lack of awareness of left-sided disability (anosognosia), neglect of the left side of visual space, and inability to recognize faces—of others or even one's own face in a mirror (prosopagnosia).

A patient with ideomotor apraxia is unable to execute movements although he understands which actions are required and has no paresis. The lesion is usually in the dominant (left) parietal lobe.

Witzelsucht (a propensity for childish jokes) has been described with frontal lobe lesions.

114 B D

Gerstmann's syndrome comprises
1 finger agnosia—an inability to indicate one's own or someone else's fingers
2 dysgraphia
3 dyscalculia
4 inability to distinguish right from left

(4) above is different from crossed laterality which is the preferential use of contralateral organs, e.g. the combination of right-handedness with left eye dominance.

115 Match each stuporous condition (A–E) with the person who described it (1–5):
A Periodic catatonia
B The motility psychosis
C Catatonia or 'tension insanity'
D Benign stupor
E Acute lethal catatonia

1 Kahlbaum
2 Hoch
3 Gjessing
4 Stauder
5 Leonhard

116 The following drugs increase fast activity on the EEG:
A chlordiazepoxide
B haloperidol
C phenobarbitone
D chlorpromazine
E phenytoin

115 A3 B5 C1 D2 E4

Stupor is a condition of psychomotor inhibition manifested by lack of speech and movement, with preserved consciousness.

The main types are depressive, catatonic, organic, psychogenic, manic and simulated.

In 1874 Kahlbaum described *tension insanity* or *catatonia*, a condition in which stupor occurred in the absence of any disease of the nervous system.

Benign stupor described by Hoch in 1921 was considered by him to be a form of manic-depressive psychosis.

Gjessing studied *periodic catatonia*, and related states of stupor or excitement to different phases of nitrogen balance.

Strauder's *acute lethal catatonia* is an acute state of stupor with pyrexia. Its nature is unclear and may be a form of schizophrenia or a viral encephalitis.

Leonhard described as separate from schizophrenia, a group of functional psychoses with a favourable outcome, which he termed 'cycloid psychoses'. There are three main types—anxiety elation psychosis, confusion psychosis and motility psychosis. These conditions tend to be bipolar—two diverse clinical pictures may occur, but not usually simultaneously. In *motility psychosis* the two opposite poles are hyperkinesia or akinesia.

Hamilton M. (ed.) (1976) *Fish's Schizophrenia*. pp. 103–5. Bristol, John Wright & Sons.

Johnson J. (1982) Stupor: its diagnosis and management. *Br. J. Hosp. Med.* **27**, 530–2.

116 A C

Barbiturates, diazepam and chlordiazepoxide cause increased fast activity on the EEG. Other anticonvulsants have little effect. Chloral hydrate also increases fast activity.

Phenothiazines, butyrophenones and tricyclic antidepressants may produce slowing on the EEG and lower the threshold for epileptic discharge.

117 For each numbered condition select the lettered symptom which is associated with it:
A apraxia of gait
B the 'gramophone symptom'
C the *signe du mirroir*
D myoclonus
E akinesia

1 Pick's disease
2 Steele–Richardson–Olszewsky syndrome
3 Normal pressure hydrocephalus
4 Alzheimer's disease
5 Creutzfeldt–Jakob disease

117 A3 B1 C4 D5 E2

The unsteadiness of gait in 'normal pressure hydrocephalus' has been termed by some as *apraxia of gait*.

Mayer-Gross has described in Pick's disease the *gramophone symptom*, the repetition with correct expression and diction of an elaborate anecdote, each time as if new.

Patients with Alzheimer's disease may sit talking to their own reflection in a mirror—the *signe du mirroir*. This may be related to an inability to recognize faces (prosopagnosia), sometimes found in this condition.

Creutzfeldt–Jakob disease is a rapidly progressing condition of dementia, *myoclonus*, extrapyramidal signs and multifocal cortical signs. Slow virus infection is the likely cause.

In Steele–Richardson–Olszewsky syndrome, or progressive supranuclear palsy, Parkinsonian signs of *akinesia* and rigidity are prominent. The cortex is relatively spared and this condition has been termed a 'subcortical dementia' in contrast to, for instance, Alzheimer's disease where the pathology is mainly cortical and clinically focal cortical signs are more prominent than extrapyramidal signs.

Organic Psychiatry: Questions 117

118 **In using the Wechsler Adult Intelligence Scale (WAIS)**
 A Vocabulary is a 'Don't Hold test'
 B verbal IQ is generally more affected by brain damage than performance IQ
 C there are altogether 11 sub-tests
 D Arithmetic is a verbal sub-test
 E deterioration indices have been used as a measure of brain damage

119 **Match each of the following conditions (A–E) with the most appropriate EEG record (1–5):**
 A petit mal
 B normality
 C subacute sclerosing panencephalitis
 D cerebral tumour
 E infantile spasms

 1 periodic bilaterally synchronous high voltage slow wave complexes
 2 delta wave focus
 3 10 c/s rhythm, maximal in the occipital and parietal regions
 4 hypsarrhythmia
 5 3 c/s 'spike and wave' discharges

118 C D E

The WAIS has 11 sub-tests as follows:

Verbal sub-tests:
1 Information
2 Comprehension
3 Arithmetic
4 Similarities
5 Digit span
6 Vocabulary

Performance sub-tests:
1 Digit symbol
2 Picture completion
3 Block design
4 Picture arrangement
5 Object assembly

Separate verbal and performance IQs can be computed, as well as a full scale IQ. A significant discrepancy between verbal and performance IQs (in favour of verbal IQ) suggests organic impairment.

Deterioration indices compare so-called 'Hold tests' (Information, Vocabulary, Picture completion and Object assembly) and 'Don't Hold tests' (Similarities, Digit span, Digit symbol and Block design). Function on 'Don't Hold tests' tends to decline early with organic impairment while ability on 'Hold tests' holds up, i.e. is more resistant to the effects of brain damage. Hence comparison of scores on 'Hold tests' and 'Don't Hold tests' might provide a measure of organic impairment.

Separate sub-tests on the WAIS in measuring different aspects of cognitive function may also provide leads to localizing brain damage, which may be pursued using other psychometric tests.

119 A5 B3 C1 D2 E4

The EEG in *infantile spasms* (salaam attacks) is characteristically disorganized—hypsarrhythmia. Spikes, sharp waves and bursts of spike and wave occur at very high voltage, randomly over both hemispheres.

The EEG complexes in *subacute sclerosing panencephalitis* typically occur at fixed intervals of 5–10 seconds synchronous with the myoclonic jerks, but may appear in the absence of any motor abnormality.

The *normal* EEG is alpha (8–13 c/s) rhythm most prominent in the occipital and parietal regions.

Three c/s spike and wave complexes characterize *petit mal* epilepsy and a space occupying lesion such as a *tumour* may produce focal slow waves on EEG.

120 The following statements concerning head injury are true:
A normal pressure hydrocephalus is a recognized sequela
B retrograde amnesia is a better guide to the severity of injury than post-traumatic amnesia
C epilepsy occurs in about 30 per cent of those with closed head injuries
D post-traumatic amnesia is a more useful measure of the severity of brain damage, in closed rather than open head injuries
E the retrograde amnesia is usually shorter than the post-traumatic amnesia

121 Activating procedures in electroencephalography include
A photic stimulation
B administration of chlorpromazine
C sleep induction
D hypoventilation
E intravenous thiopentone

120 A D E
Retrograde amnesia (RA) concerns the time between the injury and the last event before the injury which the patient can recollect. *Post-traumatic amnesia* (PTA) lasts from the time of injury to the resumption of normal uninterrupted memory. Most RAs last less than a minute and the RA is usually much shorter than the PTA.

The duration of PTA is a better guide to the severity of the injury and the prognosis for recovery than RA, and such predictions are more valid in cases of closed rather than open head injury.

Epilepsy develops in about 5 per cent of closed head injury and about 30 per cent of those with open head injury.

The aetiology of 'normal pressure hydrocephalus' is frequently unclear, but cases have been described resulting from head injury, meningitis or subarachnoid haemorrhage.

121 A B C E
With *photic stimulation,* using a flash frequency 8–15 c/s, alpha rhythm occurs synchronous with flash rate (occipital driving) and paroxysmal abnormalities including seizures may be provoked.

Drugs such as chlorpromazine, metrazole or megimide may be used to provoke seizures.

Sleep, natural or induced by barbiturates, may activate epileptic discharges, particularly those arising in the temporal lobes.

Intravenous *thiopentone* induces beta rhythm, which is, however, less prominent over areas of temporal lobe damage; hence lesions may be pinpointed.

Hyperventilation may reveal epileptic activity. Cortical excitability is thought to result from cerebral hypoxia as a result of hypocapnia-induced constriction of cerebral arterioles.

Further reading

Lishman W.A. (1978) *Organic Psychiatry.* Oxford, Blackwell Scientific Publications.
Robertson E.E. (1978) Organic disorders. In Forrest A., Affleck J. & Zealley A. (eds) *Companion to Psychiatric Studies.* pp. 459–98. Edinburgh, Churchill Livingstone.
Scott D. (1976) *Understanding E.E.G.* London, Duckworth.

Psychogeriatrics

122 The following are true of people aged over 65:
  A about 20 per cent are demented
  B they account for 14 per cent of the population of England and Wales
  C about one third of late paraphrenics have impaired hearing
  D presenile dementia occurs in about 5 per cent
  E about 10 per cent have neurotic and character disorders

123 In people over the age of 65 years
  A expression of suicidal thoughts need not be taken seriously
  B 5 per cent of all parasuicides take place
  C 10 per cent of all suicides occur
  D parasuicide is more common than suicide
  E at least a quarter of all suicides take place

124 The following are true of Pick's disease:
  A visual agnosia is an early sign
  B it is the commonest type of presenile dementia
  C females are affected more often than males
  D inheritance is by a single autosomal recessive gene
  E hyperalgesia has been described

122 B C E

In one study of the over 65 (Kay et al., 1964) about 10 per cent were demented, 3 per cent had major functional disorders and 10 per cent had neurotic and personality disorders.

An association has been demonstrated between deafness and paranoid illness in the elderly (Cooper et al., 1974). Impaired hearing occurs in about one third of late paraphrenics.

Presenile dementia by definition only occurs in those aged less than 65 years.

Cooper A.F., Curry A.R., Kay D.W.K., Garside R.F. & Roth M. (1974) Hearing loss in paranoid and affective psychoses of the elderly. Lancet **II**, 851–4.

Kay D.W.K., Beamish P. & Roth M. (1964) Old age mental disorders in Newcastle upon Tyne. Part 1: A study of prevalence. Br. J. Psychiat. **110**, 146.

123 B E

Over the age of 65 suicide is more common than parasuicide. In contrast, at younger ages the ratio of parasuicide to suicide is 10:1.

Between 25 and 30 per cent of suicides and 5 per cent of parasuicides occur in those over 65 years old.

Attempted or completed suicide is associated with depressive illness more often in the elderly than in younger people. While expression of suicidal thoughts should be taken seriously at any age, this is particularly so for the over 65s.

124 C E

Pick's disease is a rare condition, much less common than Alzheimer's disease. It affects women about twice as often as men and appears to be transmitted by an autosomal dominant gene.

Pathology involves mainly the frontal and temporal lobes, so that parietal lobe symptoms such as agnosia, apraxia and dysphasia are much less common in Pick's than in Alzheimer's disease. Frontal lobe involvement manifested by changes in social behaviour occurs at an early stage.

Hyperalgesia similar to that found in the thalamic syndrome has been described as occurring in the middle stage and diminishing as the disease progressed (Robertson et al., 1958).

Robertson E.E., Le Roux A. & Brown J.H. (1958) The clinical differentiation of Pick's disease. J. Ment. Sci. **104**, 1000–24.

Psychogeriatrics: Questions

125 The following features make a diagnosis of arteriosclerotic (multi-infarct) dementia more likely than one of senile dementia:
A personality preservation
B female sex
C gradual onset
D focal neurological signs
E hypertension

126 Match each of the following conditions (A–E) with the appropriate pathological lesion (1–5):
A Creutzfeldt–Jakob disease
B Pick's disease
C Huntington's chorea
D Alzheimer's disease
E normal pressure hydrocephalus

1 aggregates of degenerating neuronal processes around an amyloid core
2 cerebral atrophy affecting mainly the frontal lobes and caudate nucleus
3 silver-staining inclusion bodies
4 gross ventricular dilatation
5 spongiform degeneration

125 A D E

Unlike senile dementia, which more often affects women than men, multi-infarct dementia is more common in men.

Multi-infarct dementia is often associated with hypertension and the onset is acute more often than in senile dementia. It is characterized by a stepwise course with the appearance of focal neurological signs such as hemiparesis, dysphasia or dysphagia, which may recover to varying degrees. Personality preservation to a late stage of the condition is also characteristic and may be associated with a distressing insight into the decline in functioning.

126 A5 B3 C2 D1 E4

The pathology in Alzheimer's disease is of diffuse cerebral atrophy often particularly affecting the frontal and temporal lobes. Characteristically present are large numbers of neurofibrillary tangles and senile plaques (each of which consists of a collection of degenerating neuronal processes around an amyloid core).

Pick's disease 'picks out' the frontal and temporal lobes. The rest of the cortex is relatively spared. Silver-staining inclusion bodies (Pick bodies) and balloon cells are characteristic.

Cerebral atrophy in Huntington's chorea effects mainly the frontal lobes and caudate nucleus. Brain levels of γ-aminobutyric acid are decreased.

Pathological changes in Creutzfeldt–Jakob disease are a profound proliferation of astrocytes and widespread spongiform degeneration.

Symmetrical and often gross ventricular dilatation occurs in 'normal pressure hydrocephalus'.

127 The following are true of Alzheimer's disease:
   A there is an association with Down's syndrome
   B male to female ratio affected is 3 to 2
   C it usually presents with personality change
   D acetylcholinesterase activity is increased in affected brains
   E EEG abnormality is uncommon

127 A
Women are about twice as commonly affected as men. Down's syndrome individuals who live into middle age seem to be particularly prone to develop Alzheimer's disease.

Unlike Pick's disease, in which the early signs are typically personality changes attributable to frontal lobe involvement, Alzheimer's disease characteristically presents with memory impairment.

Pathological lesions are similar in Alzheimer's disease and senile dementia and there is evidence of a reduction in the activity of both choline acetyltransferase and acetylcholinesterase in brains affected by either condition. This finding provides a rationale for trials of choline and lecithin as treatment in these conditions.

The EEG is abnormal in virtually all cases with reduced alpha rhythm and increased slow activity. Grand mal fits commonly occur.

Further reading

Brandon S. (1979) The organic psychiatry of old age. In Granville-Grossman K.L. (ed.) *Recent Advances in Clinical Psychiatry*—3. pp. 135–60. Edinburgh, Churchill Livingstone.
Jacoby R.J. (1981) Depression in the elderly. *Br. J. Hosp. Med.* **25,** 40.
Levy R. & Post F. (eds) (1982) *The Psychiatry of Late Life.* Oxford, Blackwell Scientific Publications.
Post F. (1965) *The Clinical Psychiatry of Late Life.* Oxford, Pergamon Press.

Child Psychiatry

128 Specific reading retardation is associated with
   A poor concentration
   B difficulty differentiating right and left
   C precocious speech
   D a family history of reading difficulties
   E female sex
   F antisocial behaviour

129 For each of the following conditions (A–E) select the most appropriate theory of aetiology (1–5):
   A hyperkinetic syndrome
   B school refusal
   C encopresis
   D infantile autism
   E subacute sclerosing panencephalitis

   1 coercive toilet training
   2 measles virus
   3 under-aroused central nervous system
   4 separation anxiety
   5 'refrigerator' parents

128 A B D F

The term *specific reading retardation* is applicable to those children whose reading ability falls significantly below that which age, IQ and education would predict.

Boys are affected more than girls and there is frequently a family history of reading difficulties. There is an association with antisocial behaviour (see Question 130).

Other associations include spelling difficulties, *delay* in learning to speak, confusion between right and left, poorly coordinated writing, clumsiness, a lack of concentration and large family size.

129 A3 B4 C1 D5 E2

Subacute sclerosing panencephalitis is a rare condition (affecting about one child in a million in this country). Boys are affected more commonly than girls and the average age of onset is eight years. Progressive deterioration in intellectual function and behaviour, with myoclonus, leads to death within one to three years of onset. Most cases are probably due to the measles virus, and the CSF anti-measles antibody titre is often elevated. EEG is characteristic, with periodic complexes coincident with the myoclonus.

Separation anxiety appears to underlie many cases of *school refusal*, particularly in younger children. However, in some cases other mechanisms may be more significant, such as a phobia of some aspect of the school condition, or general social withdrawal which occurs typically in older children and is often associated with other depressive symptoms.

Certain cases of *encopresis* appear to reflect a disturbed child–parent relationship. The mother is often fastidious, controlling and over-concerned with cleanliness, and toilet training has been early and coercive. In this type of case soiling, particularly when associated with smearing, appears to be aggressive and often causes considerable parental irritation. Other mechanisms in encopresis include the temporary breakdown of bowel control in situations of psychological stress, a failure ever to learn bowel control, and organic conditions resulting in bowel dysfunction (and stools which appear abnormal).

Kanner (1943) suggested that the parents of children with *infantile autism* tended to be highly intelligent, rather obsessive and emotionally cool, but there is no firm evidence for this.

It has been theorized that children with the *hyperkinetic syndrome* have under-aroused central nervous systems, so that the cortex exerts relatively little inhibition over sensory input or motor output. This provides a rationale for the use of stimulants such as dextro-amphetamine and methylphenidate which may act on the reticular activating system, bringing about increased cortical inhibition.

Kanner L. (1943) Autistic disturbance of affective contact. *Nerv. Child* 2, 217–50.

Child Psychiatry: Questions

130 The following statements concerning conduct disorder are true:
  A it is the most prevalent child psychiatric disorder
  B antisocial behaviour associated with personality abnormalities is more likely to be solitary than socialized
  C delinquency is a synonymous term
  D reading retardation is significantly associated
  E prognosis is good

131 The following are characteristic of infantile autism:
  A poor understanding of speech
  B echolalia
  C hallucinations
  D poor eye-to-eye gaze
  E pronominal reversal

130 A B D

A distinction may usefully be drawn between the terms conduct disorder and delinquency. Usually regarded as a sociological description, the term delinquency is applicable to any child who infringes the law (who will be over the age of criminal responsibility which is 10 years in the UK). On the other hand, conduct disorder is a psychological description best reserved for children who not only exhibit antisocial behaviour but are also impaired with regard to personal functioning or happiness.

Conduct disorder is the most prevalent psychiatric disorder of children. The prognosis is gloomy. In a long-term follow-up of former child guidance patients Robins (1966) found that 28 per cent of antisocial children became sociopathic adults compared with only 2 per cent of a control group of normal children.

While antisocial behaviour which is unsocialized or solitary is associated with personality abnormalities, children displaying socially disapproved of behaviour in a context such as a gang tend to be normal in personality and their behaviour may be considered normal within that subcultural setting.

There appears to be a marked association between reading retardation and conduct disorders. In one study one third of 10 and 11 year olds with severe reading retardation showed antisocial behaviour, while one third of the antisocial children were severely retarded in their reading (Rutter et al., 1970).

Robins L. (1966) *Deviant Children Grown Up*. Baltimore, Williams and Wilkins.
Rutter M.L., Tizard J. & Whitmore K. (eds) (1970) *Education, Health and Behaviour*. London, Longman.

131 A B D E

Three groups of symptoms are characteristic of infantile autism:
1 Social abnormalities including a lack of attachment behaviour, poor eye-to-eye gaze, a lack of cooperative group play, failure to make friendships and a lack of empathic feeling towards others.
2 Abnormalities of language including poor comprehension, echolalia and I–You pronominal reversal (e.g. 'You want the toy' meaning 'I want the toy').
3 An insistence on sameness, for instance limited patterns of play, attachments to particular objects, unusual preoccupations and compulsive phenomena.

Certain other behaviours are common in autistic children, such as stereotyped movements, self-injury and overactivity.

Hallucinations are not a feature of infantile autism.

132 Tics
 A occur most commonly in the limbs
 B persist during sleep
 C can be suppressed voluntarily
 D are more common in boys than girls
 E occur in about 10 per cent of children at some stage

133 Enuresis occurs
 A during rapid eye movement (REM) sleep
 B more commonly in socio-economic classes 4 and 5
 C with greater concordance in monozygotic (MZ) than dizygotic (DZ) twins
 D more commonly in females than males
 E in association with other psychiatric disorders no more often than in the general child population

132 C D E

Tics are quick, sudden, coordinated but purposeless movements. They are usually facial—for instance blinking or grimacing; vocal tics may occur, manifested as grunts, or coprolalia as in Gilles de la Tourette syndrome.

Tiquers are predominantly male (male to female ratio of about 3 to 1) and perhaps 10 per cent of normal children show tic-like movements at some time.

Tics can be suppressed voluntarily but at the expense of increased tension. They disappear during sleep and often are aggravated by anxiety.

133 B C

Enuresis occurs more commonly in socio-economic classes 4 and 5, in large families and in males. There is a higher incidence in relatives and a greater concordance in MZ and DZ twins.

It seems to be associated with a small functional bladder capacity and always occurs in non-REM sleep. While the majority of enuretics are psychiatrically normal, psychiatric disorder is twice as common in enuretics as in the general population. With the exception of encopresis no specific psychiatric syndrome is particularly associated.

Kolvin I., MacKeith R. & Meadow S.R. (eds) (1973) *Bladder Control and Enuresis*. Clinics in Developmental Medicine, Nos 48/49. London, SIMP/ Heinemann.

134 The following statements are true of infantile autism:
   A visuo-spatial skill usually exceeds language skill
   B schizophrenia is the same syndrome
   C about 60 per cent of autistic children remain totally unable to live independently
   D Kanner first described the syndrome
   E onset occurs after 30 months
   F the child's IQ is a poor prognostic indicator

135 Recognized treatments of enuresis include
   A a 'bell and pad' alarm
   B imipramine
   C methylphenidate
   D a star chart
   E massed practice

134 A C D

The first description of infantile autism was by Kanner (1943). Certain symptoms are typical (see Question 131). A further characteristic appears to be an onset before the age of 30 months.

A specific cognitive deficit concerning language is present, and usually scores on tests involving language are poor compared to those on tests of visuo-spatial function.

Schizophrenia does sometimes begin in childhood when the symptomatology is similar to that seen in adults. Schizophrenia presenting in childhood and infantile autism appear to be separate conditions, differing in symptomatology, age of onset, family history, cognitive function and prognosis (Kolvin, 1971).

About 60 per cent of autistic children remain severely handicapped and totally incapable of living independently. About 1 in 6 function well in society, and the rest have an intermediate outcome. An important prognostic factor is IQ. Almost all autistic children with an IQ below 50 have a very poor outcome.

Kanner L. (1943) Autistic disturbances of affective contact. *Nerv. Child* **2**, 217–50.
Kolvin I. (1971) Psychoses in childhood—a comparative study. In Rutter M. (ed.) *Infantile Autism: Concepts, Characteristics and Treatment*. London, Churchill Livingstone.

135 A B D

Assessment of the enuretic child should include history taking, examination and urine screening for organisms, protein and glucose. Neurological disorder, urinary tract infection and diabetes mellitus should be excluded.

A simple star chart, on which the child sticks a star whenever he has a 'dry night' not only provides a baseline record of the frequency of wetting, but may be sufficient treatment in itself.

The 'bell and pad' alarm is more likely to bring about permanent cure than any other method. It usually consists of two electrodes in the form of metal sheets, separated by a cotton sheet, and linked to an alarm. When the child passes urine, electrical contact is made between the two electrodes and the bell sounds. When woken by the alarm, he should get up, switch off the alarm and empty his bladder into a chamber pot. He should then at least assist his parents in replacing the wet sheets by dry ones.

Tricyclic antidepressants such as imipramine or amitryptyline have an antieneuretic effect, but the relapse rate on discontinuing the drug is high.

Methylphenidate and massed practice are recognized treatments of the hyperkinetic syndrome and tics respectively, not of enuresis.

136 School refusal is associated with
  A at least average academic achievement
  B antisocial behaviour
  C overprotective parents
  D low social class
  E parental absence in infancy and later childhood
  F inconsistent discipline at home

136 A C
School refusal and truancy appear to be clinically distinct. Truancy is associated with below average academic attainment, other forms of antisocial behaviour and a disharmonious, lower social class family background with inconsistent parental discipline. On the other hand, school refusers seem to have had less experience of maternal absence in childhood, are dependent and overprotected and show a high standard of academic achievement and behaviour at school.

Further reading

Barker P. (1979) *Basic Child Psychiatry*. London, Granada.
Hill P. (1979) Child psychiatry. In Hill P., Murray R. & Thorley A. (eds) *Essentials of Postgraduate Psychiatry*. London, Academic Press.
Kolvin I. & MacMillan A. (1976) Child psychiatry. In Granville-Grossman K.L. (ed.) *Recent Advances in Clinical Psychiatry*—2. pp. 296-350. Edinburgh, Churchill Livingstone.
Kolvin I. & Nicol A.R. (1979) Child psychiatry. In Granville-Grossman K.L. (ed.) *Recent Advances in Clinical Psychiatry*—3. pp. 297-332. Edinburgh, Churchill Livingstone.
Kolvin I. & Goodyer I. (1982) Child psychiatry. In Granville-Grossman K.L. (ed.) *Recent Advances in Clinical Psychiatry*—4. pp. 1-24. Edinburgh, Churchill Livingstone.
Rutter M.L. & Hersov L. (eds) (1977) *Child Psychiatry: Modern Approaches*. Oxford, Blackwell Scientific Publications.
Wolkind S.N. & Coleman J.C. (1981) The psychiatry of adolescence. In Crown S. (ed.) *Practical Psychiatry*. Vol. 1. London, Northwood Books.

Mental Retardation

137 **In the assessment and treatment of the mentally handicapped the following are true:**
 A behaviour modification techniques are not applicable to the severely handicapped
 B the Gunzburg Progress Assessment Charts are a standardized test of development
 C a raised concentration of alpha-fetoprotein in the amniotic fluid is specific to open neural tube defects
 D under the Mental Health Act 1983 the term 'subnormality' has been replaced by 'retardation'
 E at present most severely subnormal children (less than 16 years old) are hospitalized

137 *All false*

Under the Mental Health Act 1983 'mental subnormality' is replaced by 'mental impairment'.

There are other causes than open spina bifida and anencephaly for an increased concentration of alpha-fetoprotein in amniotic fluid. These include bowel atresia, omphalocoele (a congenital protrusion of intestine through a defect in the abdominal wall), intra-uterine death, Turner's syndrome and congenital nephrosis.

Several scales for developmental assessment of the mentally impaired are available including the Griffith Development Scale, the Vineland Social Maturity Scale and the Gunzburg Progress Assessment Charts of Social Development. This last-mentioned method is not standardized but allows the progress of an individual subject to be followed by raters without any special training or expertise.

Behaviour modification techniques may be effectively used with the mildly and severely subnormal. Desirable patterns of behaviour may be brought about using methods of 'modelling', 'shaping' and 'prompting'. Rewards in operant conditioning programmes should be prompt.

'Time out', placement of the patient in a room on his own for a short time and hence withdrawal of positive reinforcement such as social interaction, may be employed in response to inappropriate behaviour.

Probably about 70 per cent of severely subnormal children live at home, 20 per cent are hospitalized and 10 per cent require residential care in the community.

138 Match each of the following Inborn Errors of Metabolism (A–E) to the appropriate enzyme (1–5), deficiency of which causes that condition:
A Von Gierke's disease
B homocystinuria
C Refsum's disease
D Niemann–Pick disease
E galactosaemia

1 glucose-6-phosphatase
2 sphingomyelinase
3 galactose-1-phosphate uridyl transferase
4 cystathionine synthetase
5 phytanic acid oxidase

138 A1 B4 C5 D2 E3

A useful classification of Inborn Errors of Metabolism associated with mental subnormality is as follows:

Disorders of amino-acid metabolism
1 Overflow aminoacidurias, include
  phenylketonuria
  homocystinuria
  arginosuccinic aciduria
2 Renal (transport) aminoacidurias, include
  Hartnup's disease

Disorders of carbohydrate metabolism
1 galactosaemia
2 glycogen storge diseases, include
  Von Gierke's disease

Disorders of lipid metabolism
1 Lipidoses, include
  Tay–Sachs disease
  Niemann–Pick disease
  Gaucher's disease
  metachromatic leucodystrophy
2 Refsum's disease

Disorders of connective tissue
Mucopolysaccharidosis
Type 1—Hurler's syndrome
Type 2—Hunter's syndrome
Type 3—Sanfilippo syndrome

Miscellaneous group
1 Lesch–Nyhan syndrome
2 glucose-6-phosphate dehydrogenase (G-6PD) deficiency
3 Wilson's disease (hepatolenticular degeneration)
4 hypothyroidism (cretinism)
5 nephrogenic diabetes insipidus

Mental Retardation: Questions

139 The following conditions are inherited in an X-linked manner:
A Crouzon's syndrome
B Hurler's syndrome
C Lesch–Nyhan syndrome
D nephrogenic diabetes insipidus
E Hunter's syndrome

140 The following conditions are transmitted as autosomal recessive:
A homocystinuria
B tuberous sclerosis
C Laurence–Moon–Biedl syndrome
D glucose-6-phosphatase deficiency
E all of the above

141 Match each of the following features (A–E) with the condition (1–5) in which it typically occurs:
A polydactyly
B gynaecomastia
C IgA deficiency
D phakomata
E rocker bottom feet

1 Klinefelter's syndrome
2 Laurence–Moon–Biedl syndrome
3 Edward's syndrome
4 ataxia telangiectasia
5 tuberous sclerosis

142 Match each of the following features (A–E) with the condition (1–5) in which it typically occurs:
A ichthyosis
B macular cherry-red spot
C facial naevus
D pellagra
E arachnodactyly

1 Sturge–Weber syndrome
2 Hartnup's disease
3 homocystinuria
4 Refsum's disease
5 Tay–Sachs disease

139 *C D E*

Conditions associated with mental subnormality and inherited in an X-linked manner include: Hunter's syndrome (the only type of mucopolysaccharidosis inherited in this way, the rest are transmitted as autosomal recessive), glucose-6-phosphate dehydrogenase deficiency, Lesch–Nyhan syndrome, nephrogenic diabetes insipidus, Lowe's syndrome (oculocerebro-renal syndrome, Menke's 'kinky hair' syndrome, X-linked hydrocephalus, X-linked spastic paraplegia, Norrie's disease (oculocerebral degeneration) and Renpenning's syndrome.

Hurler's syndrome (Type 1 mucopolysaccharidosis) is inherited as autosomal recessive. Crouzon's syndrome (craniofacial dysostosis) is inherited in an autosomal dominant way (see Question 140).

140 *A C D*

Glucose-6-phosphatase deficiency is Von Gierke's disease, one of the glycogen storage disorders, which are inherited as autosomal recessive.

Tuberous sclerosis is inherited as autosomal dominant. Other conditions associated with mental impairment and transmitted as autosomal dominant include: Crouzon's disease (craniofacial dysostosis), Apert's syndrome, the first arch syndromes and Greig's syndrome (hypertelorism), although this last syndrome may be transmitted also as autosomal recessive, in some families.

141 *A2 B1 C4 D5 E3*

See Heaton-Ward W.A. (1975) *Mental Subnormality*. Bristol, John Wright & Sons.

142 *A4 B5 C1 D2 E3*

See Heaton-Ward W.A. (1975) *Mental Subnormality*. Bristol, John Wright & Sons.

143 There is an increased incidence of the following in Down's syndrome:
A Hirshsprung's disease
B chronic blepharitis
C coarctation of the aorta
D lymphocytic thyroiditis
E dislocation of the lens of the eye

144 The following are recognized clinical features of Down's syndrome:
A a mewing cry
B clinodactyly
C Brushfield spots
D a large tongue
E hypertelorism

145 The following statements concerning Down's syndrome are true:
A there is a raised familial incidence when due to trisomy 21
B in cases of translocation one parent has a chromosome count of 47
C in mosaicism the body cells are all trisomic
D the overall incidence is 1 in 600
E the type due to chromosomal translocation is related to maternal age at birth

143 A B D

There is an increased incidence in Down's syndrome of septal heart defects particularly ventricular, respiratory infections, cataracts, chronic blepharitis (lysozyme which normally counters infection is absent from the tears) duodenal atresia, Hirshsprung's disease, lymphocytic thyroiditis and possibly acute leukaemia.

Coarctation of the aorta is excessively frequent in Turner's and Marfan's syndromes, and lens dislocation in Marfan's syndrome (typically upward dislocation) and homocystinuria (usually downward dislocation).

144 B C

Recognized features of Down's syndrome are severe subnormality, a small round head (brachycephaly), a mongoloid slant to the palpebral fissures, epicanthic folds, white speckling of the iris (Brushfield spots), a tongue which protrudes and has transverse furrows but is not usually larger than normal, a short thick neck, small stature, short limbs, hypotonia, a transverse crease of the palm (simian crease), short fingers, and incurving of the fifth finger (clinodactyly). The dermatoglyphic pattern including a large 'a t d' angle is pathognomonic.

Hypertelorism and a mewing cry are features of the *cri du chat* syndrome.

145 D

There are three kinds of genotypal disorder in Down's syndrome:

1 *Trisomy 21*, which results from non-dysjunction. Although the extra chromosome has now been identified by fluorescent banding techniques as a chromosome 22 and not 21 as originally thought, for convenience the original nomenclature is retained. Affected individuals have 47 chromosomes. This kind of Down's syndrome is related to maternal age. A mother who has such a child is *not* at greater risk of producing another child similarly affected than any other woman of the same age. Familial incidence is *not* increased.

2 *Translocation*, in which the extra chromosome is fused to another (see Question 147) so that the number of chromosomes appears to be 46. This disorder is usually inherited and 'carrier' parents and siblings occur having the translocation chromosome and an apparent total chromosome number of 45. The incidence of Down's syndrome due to translocation is unrelated to maternal age.

3 *Mosaicism*. Normal cells coexist with trisomic cells in the body. Non-dysjunction after fertilization is thought to be the causal mechanism.

146 The following statements are true of phenylketonuria:
A phenylpyruvic acid is excreted in the urine
B the Guthrie test should be carried out in the first three days
C incidence is 1 in 12 000 live births
D treatment is with a phenylalanine-free diet
E brain damage is present at birth in those homozygous for the phenylketonuric gene

147 Match each of the following genotypes (A–F) with the corresponding clinical condition (1–6):
A deletion of short arm of chromosome 5
B translocation 15/21
C trisomy 13–15
D deletion of short arm of chromosome 4
E XXY
F trisomy 17–18

1 Edward's syndrome
2 Wolf's syndrome
3 Patau's syndrome
4 Klinefelter's syndrome
5 *cri du chat* syndrome
6 Down's syndrome

148 The following conditions are more common in the mentally retarded:
A autism
B manic-depressive psychosis
C epilepsy
D hysterical conversion
E hyperkinetic syndrome

146 *A C*

This condition results from a deficiency of the enzyme phenylalanine hydroxylase, which converts phenylalanine to tyrosine. As a consequence of the deficiency phenylalanine accumulates in the blood and phenylpyruvic acid is excreted in the urine.

A commonly used screening test for raised levels of blood phenylalanine is the Guthrie test. This quantitative procedure depends on the ability of phenylalanine to promote the growth of Bacillus subtilis in the presence of an inhibitory substance in the culture medium. Blood may be obtained by a heel prick and the test should be carried out between six and 14 days of age for valid results. Testing before six days may give misleadingly high levels in females.

Infants homozygous for the phenylketonuric trait are not brain-damaged at birth and only become so when they ingest phenylalanine.

Mental impairment may be prevented in affected children by providing from birth a diet in which phenylalanine is not absent, but restricted in amount. If phenylalanine intake is insufficient anorexia, diarrhoea, an eczematous rash, physical and mental retardation may occur in the child. Serum levels of phenylalanine should be maintained between 4 and 8 mg per 100 ml.

147 *A5 B6 C3 D2 E4 F1*

Chromosome pairs have been grouped as follows: pairs 1 to 3, Group A; pairs 4 to 5, Group B; pairs 6 to 12, Group C; pairs 13 to 15, Group D; pairs 16 to 18, Group E; pairs 19 to 20, Group F; and pairs 21 and 22, Group G, plus a pair of sex chromosomes. So, alternative names for Patau's syndrome (trisomy 13–15) and Edward's syndrome (trisomy 17–18) are trisomy D and trisomy E respectively.

In the type of Down's syndrome due to translocation, the extra chromosome (21) becomes fused to a member of another chromosome pair to produce a 13/21, 14/21, 15/21, 21/21 or 21/22 translocation (see also Question 145).

148 *A C D E*

Hysterical conversion symptoms and epilepsy are held to be more prevalent and manic-depressive psychosis less common in the mentally retarded.

Psychiatric disorder (conduct disorder and emotional disorder) is more common in intellectually retarded children (Rutter *et al.*, 1970).

Autism and hyperkinetic syndrome are associated with severe intellectual retardation. In the case of autism, as many as 70 per cent of affected children have IQs less than 70 and 40 per cent IQs below 50.

Rutter M., Tizard J. & Whitmore K. (1970) *Education, Health and Behaviour.* London, Longman.

149

The following statements concerning mental retardation are true (an IQ less than 50 is roughly equivalent to *severe* retardation and an IQ of 50 to 70 roughly equivalent to *mild* retardation):

A parents of the mildly retarded are mainly from the lower social classes
B phenylketonuria is the commonest specific cause of mental retardation
C with the diagnostic methods now available, a specific pathological cause is detectable in most cases of mental retardation
D parents of the mildly retarded tend to be more intelligent than those of the severely retarded
E individuals with Down's sydrome tend to be more aggressive than others with mental retardation

150

The following statements are true of Piaget's stages of intellectual development:

A a four-year-old child is egocentric
B the sensorimotor stage occurs between the ages of seven and 12 years
C a child thinks in abstract terms before attaining the concept of object permanence
D a child separates himself mentally from objects during the first two years
E conservation concepts are normally achieved by the age of 12 years

149 A

A specific pathological cause is not identifiable for the majority of mentally retarded individuals. For most (the subcultural group), the impairment is the consequent of a combination of genetic and environmental factors.

Specific disease processes are more likely to be found in the severely retarded. Down's syndrome, meningitis and phenylketonuria (in that order) are the commonest specific conditions associated with mental retardation.

While parents of those with mild retardation are predominantly lower social class and tend to be below average in intelligence, parents of the severely retarded are more evenly distributed with respect to social class and intelligence.

Individuals with Down's syndrome tend to be less aggressive and antisocial than other mentally retarded people. (Those with phenylketonuria are generally more aggressive than others with mental retardation.)

150 A D E

Piaget described four stages of cognitive development:

1 *Sensorimotor*, from birth to two years of age, during which a child begins to *differentiate himself* from the external world. The concept of *object permanence* (a belief that objects exist even when not perceived) develops.

2 *Pre-operational* (between two and seven years). A child's behaviour is influenced by concepts of *egocentrism*, animism, pre-causal logic, authoritarian morality and irreversibility. He begins to achieve *conservation concepts*, first for number (at about six years), then mass (at age of seven) and later for weight (at about nine years).

3 *Concrete operational* (seven to 12 years). The capacity for logical thought develops.

4 *Formal operational* (12 years and over). *Abstract or symbolic thought* and the ability to hypothesize occur.

There is experimental support for the sequence of intellectual development as described by Piaget; however, there appears to be great individual variation in the ages at which the various stages are reached.

Hilgard E.R., Atkinson R.C. & Atkinson R.L. (1975) *Introduction to Psychology*. pp. 75–8. New York, Harcourt Brace.

Further reading

Department of Health and Social Security, Welsh Office (1971) *Better Services for the Mentally Handicapped*. London, Her Majesty's Stationery Office.

Heaton-Ward W.A. (1975) *Mental Subnormality*. Bristol, John Wright & Sons.

Forensic Psychiatry

150 **The following statements concerning juvenile delinquency are true:**
A delinquents are more likely than non-delinquents to have criminal fathers
B it is associated with discord within the family
C 10 per cent of all indictable crime is committed by individuals under 21 years of age
D twin studies have demonstrated clearly a higher concordance rate in monozygotic (MZ) as compared to dizygotic (DZ) pairs
E there is an association with large family size

151 **The following are terms defined in the Mental Health Act 1983:**
A mental handicap
B severe subnormality
C mental disorder
D psychopathic disorder
E severe mental impairment

152 **A homosexual act is**
A illegal if one partner is 15 years old
B always lawful between consenting adults
C illegal if one participant is a merchant seaman
D legal between 18 year olds, in private
E illegal if one participant is a member of Her Majesty's Services

150 *A B E*
Delinquency means behaviour which breaks the law (see Question 130). It is an important subject because of the extent of the problem (in large cities one boy in five will be convicted by the age of 21 years) and because of the severity of the offences (half of all indictable crime is committed by individuals less than 21 years of age).

Unlike studies on criminality in adults in which the concordance rate has been higher for MZ as compared to same sex DZ twins, for juvenile delinquency little if any difference has been shown between MZ and DZ twins.

Large family and family discord are associated factors, as is criminality in the fathers.

151 *C D E*
Definitions given under section 1 of the act are as follows:
Mental disorder means mental illness, arrested or incomplete development of mind, psychopathic disorder or any other disorder or disability of mind.

Severe mental impairment means a state of arrested or incomplete development of mind which includes *severe* impairment of intelligence and social functioning and is associated with abnormally aggressive or seriously irresponsible conduct on the part of the person concerned.

Mental impairment means a state of arrested or incomplete development of mind which includes *significant* impairment of intelligence and social functioning and is associated with abnormally aggressive or seriously irresponsible conduct on the part of the person concerned.

Psychopathic disorder means a persistent disorder or disability of mind (whether or not including significant impairment of intelligence) which results in abnormally aggressive or seriously irresponsible conduct on the part of the person concerned.

A person may not be regarded as suffering from mental disorder by reason only of *promiscuity or other immoral conduct, sexual deviancy or dependence on alcohol or drugs.*

152 *A C E*
According to the Sexual Offences Act 1967, which followed the Wolfenden Committee of 1958, homosexual relationships between consenting males are lawful when both parties are over 21 and when the behaviour occurs in a private place. It is not permitted if one of the participants is a member of Her Majesty's Services or the merchant navy. Homosexual acts with those who are mentally handicapped are also excluded.

153 The following statements are now true of shoplifters:
A most are female
B about 20 per cent are mentally disordered
C shoplifting may be the earliest symptom of depression
D the majority are young people
E about 10 per cent of first offenders are reconvicted

154 The following statements are true of sexual offences:
A they constitute approximately 10 per cent of all convictions
B intercourse with a girl under the age of 13 is always an offence
C most exhibitionists are reconvicted
D it is illegal for a woman over the age of 16 to allow her father to have sexual intercourse with her
E fifteen per cent of convicted sex offenders suffer from mental handicap

155 The following statements are true of paedophilia:
A the adult is usually previously unknown to the child
B the child may actively participate in two-thirds of cases
C middle-aged paedophiles are usually unmarried
D coitus is uncommon
E the peak age for girl partners is 12 to 15

153 C D E

The majority of shoplifters are aged between 10 and 18 and more are male than female. However, a recognized group is those middle-aged British women often with numerous physical complaints in whom shoplifting may be an early symptom of depression. Probably about 5 per cent of shoplifters have a psychiatric disorder.

Gibbens T.C.N. (1981) Shoplifting. *Br. J. Psychiat.* **138**, 346–7.

154 B D

Sex offences represent approximately 0.6 per cent of all convictions and 3 per cent of all indictable convictions. Only 3 per cent of convicted sex offenders suffer from mental handicap.

Intercourse with girls under the age of 16 is illegal even if consent is given; their consent is invalid. However, under the law there are two classes of offence:
1 Intercourse with a girl under the age of 13 is considered a grave offence, ranking with rape.
2 Intercourse with a girl between 13 and 16 years of age, unless by force and against her will, in which case it will be rape, is a less grave offence. Furthermore there may be a valid defence to this charge if it is demonstrated that the accused man was under 24 years old, genuinely believed and had reasonable cause to believe that the girl was over 16 years old and he had never before been charged with a similar offence.

With regard to incest, under the Sexual Offences Act 1956 it is an offence for a man to have sexual intercourse with a woman he knows to be his daughter, grand-daughter, mother, sister or half-sister and for a woman over 16 to allow a man she knows to be her son, father, grandfather, brother or half-brother, to have sexual intercourse with her. Sibling relationships are probably the most frequent type of incest, although father–daughter incest is the most commonly reported.

Generally the prognosis for convicted exhibitionists is good and most are not charged again after their first offence.

155 B D

Paedophiles are of three main types: the emotionally and sexually immature adolescent, the middle-aged man with marital problems, and the socially isolated elderly man.

The usual age range for girl partners is 6 to 11 years and for boys 12 to 15 years. The adult is usually previously known to the child and in as many as two-thirds of cases the child may actively participate, in what is usually kissing and caressing. Coitus is unusual.

Gibbens T.C.N. & Prince J. (1965) *Child Victims of Sex Offences*. London, Institute for the Study and Treatment of Delinquency.

Forensic Psychiatry: Questions 153

156 The following are true for Admission for Assessment under the Mental Health Act 1983:
A application can only be made by a relative
B the recommendation of a Section 12 approved doctor is required
C the patient may only apply to a Mental Health Review Tribunal after 14 days admission
D the nearest relative may discharge the patient
E legal requirements are given under Section 3 of the Act

157 The following statements concerning fitness to plead are true:
A the ability to examine a witness is required
B it is decided by a jury if the issue is raised
C if the issue is raised by the prosecution the case must be proved beyond reasonable doubt
D it requires the ability to instruct counsel
E a person judged unfit to plead is sent to prison

158 The following are true of the 47 XYY karyotype:
A there is an increased likelihood of criminal conviction
B physical appearance is abnormal
C the prevalence rate in British special hospitals is about 3 per cent
D tall stature is associated
E intellectual level is lower than that of XY control subjects

Forensic Psychiatry: Answers

156 B D

Section 3 refers to Admission for Treatment.

Under Section 2—Admission for Assessment, application may be made by the nearest relative or an approved social worker. The application must be supported by two medical recommendations (one of them from a Section 12 approved doctor). The patient has the right to apply to a Mental Health Review Tribunal *within* 14 days of admission. The nearest relative, the managers or the responsible medical officer (RMO) can discharge the patient, although the RMO can bar discharge by the nearest relative.

157 A B C D

Fitness to plead concerns the defendant's sanity at the time of the trial. A trial of fitness to plead is held in front of a separate jury and if considered unfit to plead a person is admitted to a special hospital until fit to plead, as decided by the Home Secretary.

Fitness to plead assumes the ability to
1 understand the charge and the significance of his plea
2 challenge a juror
3 instruct counsel
4 examine a witness
5 follow the progress of the trial

When the issue is raised by the prosecution or by the judge the case must be proved beyond reasonable doubt; however, if raised by the defendant judgement is made on the balance of probabilities.

158 A C D E

The prevalence of the XYY karyotype in special hospitals (of about 3 per cent) appears to be higher than that in subnormality hospitals and in ordinary prisons, where it seems to be higher than in the general population.

Tall stature and lower intelligence are associated, as is an increase in the likelihood of criminal conviction, although the crimes committed are probably not particularly violent ones.

There are no characteristic abnormalities in physical appearance.

Witkin H.A., Medrick S.A. & Schulsinger F. (1976) Criminality in XYY and XXY men. *Science* **193**, 547–55.

159 Under the Mental Health Act 1983 the patient's consent is always necessary for
A ECT
B implantation of hormones to reduce male sex drive
C subcaudate tractotomy
D fluphenazine injections
E stereotactic amygdalotomy

160 A person with a 'sound disposing mind' (testamentary capacity) must
A express himself clearly
B be of more than subnormal intelligence
C know the extent of his property
D know which persons have a claim on his property
E be free of delusions

161 The following are associated with non-accidental injury to children:
A low social class parents
B mothers of subnormal intelligence
C older maternal age
D unmarried mothers
E socially isolated families

162 Under Section 5(4)—Nurses Holding Power of the Mental Health Act 1983
A all state registered nurses have the authority to detain patients
B nurses are allowed to admit patients to hospital
C patients may be detained for up to 12 hours
D patients may only be held if it is not immediately possible for a doctor to implement Section 5(2)
E the patient detained must appear to have a mental disorder

159 B C E

Section 57—Treatment Requiring Consent *and* a Second Opinion, specifies certain treatments which may only be given with the consent of the patient (detained or not detained). These are, (a) any surgical operation for destroying brain tissue or for destroying the function of brain tissue, and (b) such other forms of treatment as may be specified by the Secretary of State in Regulations (so far specified is 'the surgical implantation of hormones to reduce male sexual drive').

Regulations concerning the administration of ECT or depot neuroleptics to detained patients are given under Section 58—Treatment Requiring Consent *or* a Second Opinion.

160 A C D

To make a will a person should know the nature and extent of his property, which persons have a claim on it, be able to assess the relative strengths of those claims and express himself legibly and unambiguously.

A person may be deluded, of subnormal intelligence, or even demented (depending on the complexity of the will in question) and still have a 'sound disposing mind'.

161 A B D E

It is infants who are particularly at risk of non-accidental injury. There is a tendency for the mothers of battered children to be young, unmarried and of subnormal intelligence. Personality abnormality and criminality are excessively prevalent in the fathers. The families tend to be of low social class and socially isolated, and the parents have frequently themselves been victims of non-accidental injury as children.

Scott P.D. (1977) Non-accidental injury in children. *Br. J. Psychiat.* **131**, 366–80.
Smith S.M., Hanson R. & Noble S. (1973) Parents of battered babies: a controlled study. *Br. Med. J.* **IV**, 388–91.

162 D E

This section permits registered mental nurses or registered nurses for mental handicap to detain a patient already receiving treatment for mental disorder in hospital, for up to 6 hours while a doctor is found. It must appear to the nurses that, (a) the patient is suffering from mental disorder to such a degree that it is necessary for his health or safety, or for the protection of others, for him to be immediately restrained from leaving hospital, and (b) that it is not practicable to secure the immediate attendance of a practitioner to implement Section 5(2).

Forensic Psychiatry: Questions

163 The majority of murderers
  A have lower socio-economic backgrounds
  B are middle aged
  C choose strangers as victims
  D have schizophrenia
  E are male

164 For each numbered form of psychiatric defence select the lettered answer that most closely corresponds to it:
  A 'balance of her mind was disturbed ... by ... the effects of giving birth or by ... lactation consequent upon the birth'
  B 'under disability'
  C 'labouring under such a defect of reason, from disease of the mind, as not to know the nature and quality of the act he was doing or, if he did know it, that he did not know he was doing what was wrong'
  D hypoglycaemia
  E 'such abnormality of mind ... as substantially impaired his mental responsibility for his acts and omissions in doing or being a party to the killing'

  1 not guilty by reason of insanity
  2 incapacity to form an intent (automatism)
  3 diminished responsibility
  4 infanticide
  5 unfit to plead

163 A E

Murder is unlawful killing with malice aforethought *(mens rea)*. In Britain murderers are usually young adult males from lower socio-economic backgrounds. In most cases the victims are previously known to the murderer, and female. Almost 50 per cent of murderers have a mental abnormality, particularly personality disorders, subnormality and schizophrenia.

Driver M.V., West L.R. & Faulk M. (1974) Clinical and EEG studies of prisoners charged with murder. *Br. J. Psychiat.* **125,** 583-7.

164 A4 B5 C1 D2 E3

A psychiatric defence may be entered in any of the five ways above.

A defendant considered *unfit to plead* is admitted to a special hospital where he is regarded as 'under disability' (see Question 157).

Hypoglycaemia, concussion and epilepsy are the usual conditions on which a defence on the grounds of *automatism* is based.

Not guilty by reason of insanity based on the McNaughton rules is now much less used as a defence in murder cases, since the 1957 Homicide Act and the abolition of capital punishment. This verdict results in the defendant being admitted to a hospital, usually a special hospital until a time of release decided by the Home Secretary.

A defence on the grounds of *diminished responsibility* (Homicide Act 1957) can only be used if the charge is murder and if upheld results in a verdict of guilty of manslaughter.

A woman who kills her child within one year of its birth may be found guilty of *infanticide* in which case she is dealt with as if guilty of manslaughter.

165 In non-accidental injury to children the following are typical injuries:
A fractured scaphoid bone
B subdural haematoma
C fractured neck of femur
D ruptured spleen
E subperiosteal bleeding

165 B D E

Characteristic non-accidental injuries to children are multiple bruises, burns or lacerations; separation of fragments from the metaphyses and the separation of periosteum from the shafts of bones with subperiosteal bleeding; multiple fractures; subdural haematomata; rupture of abdominal viscera.

Delay in reporting and contradictory histories of the injury should arouse suspicion.

Further reading

Bluglass R. (1979) Incest. *Br. J. Hosp. Med.* **22**, 152–7.
Gunn J. (1979) Forensic psychiatry. In Granville-Grossman K. (ed.) *Recent Advances in Clinical Psychiatry*—3. Edinburgh, Churchill Livingstone.
Hamilton J.R. (1983) The Mental Health Act, 1983. *Br. Med. J.***286**, 1720–5.
Hill P. (1979) Forensic psychiatry. In Hill P., Murray R. & Thorley A. (eds) *Essentials of Postgraduate Psychiatry.* pp. 531–67. London, Academic Press.
Her Majesty's Stationery Office (1983) *Mental Health Act 1983.* London, HMSO.
Rooth F.G. (1971) Indecent exposure and exhibitionism. *Br. J. Hosp. Med.* **6**, 521–33.
Trick K.L.K. & Tennant T.G. (1981) *Forensic Psychiatry: An Introductory Text.* London, Pitman.

Transcultural Psychiatry

166 The International Pilot Study of Schizophrenia demonstrated that
A any international differences in outcome were insignificant
B it was impossible to make valid comparisons of psychopathology in different cultures
C prevalence of schizophrenia was higher in developed countries
D psychiatrists can reliably rate symptoms in different cultural settings
E outcome was more favourable in India than in Europe

167 The following are typical features of Koro:
A occurrence in China
B fear of 'evil eye'
C suicidal behaviour
D female sex affected
E obsessions

168 Characteristic features of Piblokto are
A an overwhelming desire to eat human flesh
B amnesia for the episode
C occurrence in Eskimos
D depressed mood
E occurrence during a time of food shortage

166 D E

The International Pilot Study of Schizophrenia (World Health Organisation, 1973) was a study of the prevalence, symptomatology, course and outcome of schizophrenia in nine different countries. The Present State Examination (PSE), translated into local languages, permitted reliable psychiatric assessment in different cultures. While prevalence, using PSE assessments, was similar in all countries studied, outcome was found to be more favourable in developing as compared to developed countries, particularly for those cases with an insidious onset. The reasons for this are unclear.

World Health Organisation (1973) *The International Pilot Study of Schizophrenia.* Vol. 1. Geneva, WHO.

167 A

Certain culture-bound syndromes have been described. The effect of culture on psychiatric disorder appears to be more pathoplastic than pathogenic and the culture-bound syndromes may be mostly considered as variants of the traditional categories of psychosis or neurosis.

Koro, considered to be an acute anxiety state, affects Chinese men. They believe their penis is retracting into the abdomen and that death will ensue. The subject may attempt to prevent this by, for instance, tying string around the penis. The syndrome often occurs in the context of guilt about sexual behaviour.

Susto is another anxiety reaction described in Latin America. The subject believes that he has been changed in some way, perhaps as a result of magical substances entering his body, or because of 'evil eye'—the magical gaze of someone else.

Shinkeishitsu is an obsessional neurosis reported in young Japanese men. It may arise as a result of the high demands and expectations of life in modern technological Japan.

168 B C D

Piblokto occurs in Eskimo women. After a period of depressive brooding, in a state of dissociation they run into the snow and jump into water. Typically amnesia occurs for the episode.

Windigo is a depressive disorder reported in Canadian Indians and occurring often during periods of starvation. Cannibalistic behaviour is attributed by the subject to control by a spirit called the 'windigo'.

169 Latah is characterized by
  A echolalia
  B a response to a stressful situation
  C homicidal behaviour
  D occurrence in the Far East and Africa
  E the male sex being affected

169 A B D

Latah, regarded as an hysterical illness, affects usually females in a stressful situation. It has been reported under different names in the Far East and parts of Africa. Typically subjects are highly suggestible and show echolalia, echopraxia and automatic obedience.

Amok is a dissociative or depressive state during which subjects, nearly always men, may violently attack others. Homicidal or suicidal behaviour may occur. It has been described in South-East Asia.

Further reading

Lipsedge M. & Littlewood R. (1979) Transcultural psychiatry. In Granville-Grossman K.L. (ed.). *Recent Advances in Clinical Psychiatry*—3. pp. 91–134. Edinburgh, Churchill Livingstone.

Stein M.D. (1979) *An Introduction to Transcultural Psychiatry*. London, SK & F Publications.

Physical Methods of Treatment

170 The following statements concerning lithium therapy are true:
A the drug is partially metabolized in the liver
B lithium-induced hypothyroidism can only be treated by stopping the drug
C full benefit may not be evident before six months of treatment
D thiazide diuretics reduce lithium serum levels
E secretion of antidiuretic hormone (ADH) may be reduced leading to polyuria and polydipsia

171 Amphetamines
A release catecholamines into the synapse
B may be of benefit in the hyperkinetic syndrome
C block postsynaptic receptors
D block re-uptake of catecholamines into presynaptic neurones
E may lead to persecutory delusions

170 C

Lithium is an element; hence it cannot be destroyed, only eliminated. Renal disease, heart disease, low fluid intake, old age and thiazide diuretics may all reduce the kidney's capacity to eliminate lithium. Consequently thiazide diuretic may *increase* the serum level of lithium.

The full benefit of lithium in the prophylaxis of affective illness may not be seen before six to 12 months of treatment.

Hypothyroidism, a recognized side-effect, can be treated with thyroxine, without stopping lithium therapy.

Signs of diabetes insipidus, such as polyuria and polydipsia, may arise as side-effects of lithium therapy. This is a *nephrogenic* diabetes insipidus, and reflects a lack of responsiveness of the renal distal tubules and collecting ducts to ADH, which is secreted in normal amounts by the posterior pituitary. (*Cranial* diabetes insipidus is associated with a deficiency of ADH.)

171 *A B D E*

Amphetamines increase availability of catecholamines to postsynaptic receptors, by releasing them directly into the synaptic cleft, and by blocking their re-uptake.

Stimulant drugs such as amphetamines and methylphenidate have beneficial effects in the hyperkinetic syndrome. While anorexia, insomnia and tearfulness are common side-effects with both drugs, methylphenidate probably has less effect on height gain than dextro-amphetamine and may be preferred for this reason.

The amphetamine psychosis (Connell, 1958) is most frequently associated with prolonged high dose consumption of the drug. Visual, tactile and auditory hallucinations, ideas of reference and persecutory delusions can occur in clear consciousness so that the syndrome may be indistinguishable from paranoid schizophrenia.

Connell P.H. (1958) *Amphetamine Psychosis*. Maudsley Monograph No. 5. Oxford, Oxford University Press.

Physical Methods of Treatment: Questions

172 The following are true of electroconvulsive therapy (ECT):
   A   convulsions must be electrically induced for any therapeutic effect
   B   in most cases of chronic schizophrenia ECT brings about significant improvement
   C   the strength of the electrical stimulus is related to the degree of memory disturbance
   D   clinical trials have demonstrated the efficacy of ECT as a treatment for mania
   E   convulsive activity is necessary for therapeutic effect

173 The following statements concerning major tranquillizers are true:
   A   some endocrine side-effects of chlorpromazine are attributable to decreased levels of circulating prolactin
   B   pimozide may be of particular value in monosymptomatic hypochondriacal psychosis
   C   depot injections have reduced the incidence of drug defaulting
   D   phenothiazines block dopamine receptors on the postsynaptic membrane
   E   maintenance therapy in schizophrenia is associated with a reduced relapse rate

172 C E

There is evidence that while convulsive activity in the brain is necessary for a therapeutic effect, the strength of the electrical stimulus is related to the amount of memory disturbance. Therefore the minimum stimulus capable of inducing a convulsion should probably be used.

Whether the convulsion is induced electrically (ECT) or by some other means, e.g. photostimulation or fluorothyl inhalation, does not appear to be important for therapeutic outcome.

Although ECT has been widely used in the past for the treatment of mania, no clinical trial has been carried out to demonstrate its efficacy in this condition.

The available evidence points to ECT being of little value in *chronic* schizophrenia. In *acute* schizophrenia its efficacy is unclear; certainly with courses of up to 12 ECT treatments any beneficial effect appears to be short-lived.

173 B C D E

Dopamine appears to inhibit prolactin secretion. Phenothiazines block dopamine receptors and bring about increased circulating prolactin. Galactorrhoea, breast engorgement and amenorrhoea, which are recognized side-effects of chlorpromazine, may be attributable to hyperprolactinaemia.

Monosymptomatic hypochondriacal psychosis is a condition characterized by a single hypochondriacal delusion. There is some evidence that pimozide, which is a diphenylbutylpiperidine compound, may be of benefit in this condition.

Depot injections have increased compliance with medication. Reasons for drug defaulting include unpleasant side-effects of medication, poor communication between the prescribing doctor and the patient, the patient's attitude to the use of drugs in his illness which is particularly relevant with psychiatric illnesses, losing contact with the psychiatric services through geographical drifting, and refusal of injections.

Maintenance therapy in schizophrenia, usually with fluphenazine decanoate or flupenthixol decanoate does reduce relapse rate. Whether all schizophrenics should receive maintenance therapy and how long therapy should be continued are as yet unclear.

174 The following are true of psychosurgery:
A schizophrenia is the main indication
B Moniz devised the standard prefrontal leucotomy
C stereotactic methods have been associated with fewer unwanted side-effects
D worldwide consensus now exists concerning the optimal target sites in particular conditions
E obsessional ruminations are a contraindication

175 Unilateral non-dominant electroconvulsive therapy (ECT) has the following advantages to bilateral ECT:
A less memory disturbance occurs as a side-effect
B fewer treatments are required
C a bilateral convulsion is not necessary
D it produces less post-ictal confusion
E it gives quicker results

Physical Methods of Treatment: Answers

174 C

The Portuguese neurologist, Egaz Moniz, was a pioneer of psychosurgery. However, two American surgeons, Freeman and Watts, modified his procedure and devised the standard prefrontal leucotomy.

Complications of psychosurgery include disinhibition, lethargy and epilepsy. Although contemporary stereotactic methods have fewer complications, consensus is lacking regarding the specificity of many of the surgical approaches.

Affective disorders and obsessional neurosis are now the prime indications.

175 A D

Unilateral ECT to the non-dominant hemisphere produces less amnesia and post-ictal confusion than bilateral ECT and by the end of treatment efficacy appears to be as good.

Unilateral ECT may take a little longer to act than bilateral ECT and, on average, less than one extra treatment may be required in a typical course.

With both unilateral and bilateral ECT it should be the aim to produce a generalized rather than a focal fit. Evidence points to focal convulsions being less effective.

176 The following statements concerning the metabolism of the monoamines in the brain are true:
A tyrosine is the dietary precursor of the catecholamines
B the main central nervous system metabolite of noradrenaline is homovanillic acid
C the rate limiting step in 5-hydroxytryptamine synthesis involves tryptophan hydroxylase
D 5-hydroxytryptamine is metabolized by catechol o-methyl transferase
E dopamine β hydroxylase converts dopamine to adrenaline

176 A C

Tyrosine is the precursor of the catecholamines dopamine (DA) and noradrenaline (NA). Tyrosine hydroxylase converts it to dihydroxyphenylalanine (DOPA), which is decarboxylated to DA. NA (not adrenaline) arises from the metabolism of DA by dopamine β hydroxylase. Both DA and NA are broken down by monoamine oxidase (MAO) and catechol o-methyl transferase (COMT) to homovanillic acid (HMA) and 3-methoxy-4-hydroxyphenylglycol (MHPG) respectively.

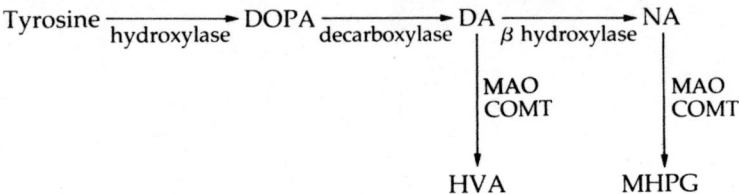

Tryptophan, the precursor amino acid of 5-hydroxytryptamine (5-HT) is hydroxylated, in a rate limiting step, to 5-hydroxytryptophan (5-HTP), which is decarboxylated to 5-HT. Breakdown of 5-HT is by MAO to 5-hydroxyindoleacetaldehyde (5-HIA). 5-hydroxyindoleacetic acid (5-HIAA) is the end produce of 5-HT metabolism in the brain.

tryptophan $\xrightarrow[\text{hydroxylase}]{}$ 5-HTP $\xrightarrow[\text{decarboxylase}]{}$ 5-HT $\xrightarrow[\text{MAO}]{}$ 5-HIA $\longrightarrow$ 5-HIAA

Physical Methods of Treatment: Questions

177 Tricyclic antidepressants
- A relieve depressive symptoms to some degree in all patients
- B should be stopped as soon as the patient has recovered from depression
- C in therapeutic doses may affect the ECG of patients without cardiac disease
- D cause an increased liability to convulsions
- E may precipitate acute retention of urine in the elderly male

178 The following are contraindications to electroconvulsive therapy (ECT):
- A an indwelling cardiac pacemaker
- B raised intracranial pressure
- C old age
- D pregnancy
- E hypochondriasis

177 C D E

Unfortunately some patients do not respond to tricyclic antidepressants—depressive symptoms are relieved in only 60 to 80 per cent of patients.

Present evidence suggests that antidepressants should not be stopped immediately after recovery from an episode of depression, but should be continued for at least six months, as this is associated with reduced risk of relapse (Mindham et al., 1973).

Cardiac effects of tricyclic drugs include tachycardia, postural hypotension and heart block. Prolonged QT, ST depression and T wave flattening may be produced on the ECG of people without cardiac disease.

Central nervous system effects include a fine tremor, ataxia, an increased liability to convulsions and a toxic confusional state.

Many of the side-effects are clearly due to anticholinergic effects, such as dry mouth, blurred vision, constipation, the precipitation of glaucoma, and also acute urinary retention in males with enlarged prostate glands.

Mindham R.H.S., Howland C. & Shepherd M. (1973) An evaluation of continuation therapy with tricyclic antidepressants in depressive illness. *Psychol. Med.* **3,** 5–17.

178 B

ECT is associated with a brief but considerable increase in cerebral blood flow and should be avoided in anyone suspected of having raised intracranial pressure.

It does not interfere with cardiac pacemakers or precipitate labour, and its effectiveness seems to be at least as good in the elderly as in younger people.

In scales which claim to predict clinical response to ECT in depression (e.g. Hobson, 1953), generally features of 'endogenous' depression, such as acute onset, retardation, early morning waking and weight loss, are considered favourable, while the reverse holds for signs of neurotic disturbance or personality disorder. Hypochondriasis has been associated with a poor response, but is not a contraindication to ECT.

Hobson R.F. (1953) Prognostic factors in electric convulsive therapy. *J. Neurol. Neurosurg. Psychiat.* **16,** 275.

179 **The following are true for patients on monoamine oxidase inhibitors (MAOIs):**
   A the effects of hypoglycaemic agents are increased
   B foodstuffs which contain tryptamine should be avoided
   C pethidine is a safer compound than morphine
   D cough mixtures may be dangerous
   E a hypertensive crisis may be treated with intravenous phentolamine

180 **Thioridazine *differs* from chlorpromazine in the following respects:**
   A it has a piperazine side chain
   B extrapyramidal effects are less common
   C retinal pigmentation is more likely
   D it blocks dopamine receptors
   E jaundice is more common

179 A D E

Tyramine (not tryptamine) is an indirect sympathomimetic amine, i.e. its effects are not by direct action on adrenergic receptors, but by provoking the release of catecholamines. Normally monoamine oxidases neutralize the effects of tyramine in the gut and the liver. MAOIs will block this protective mechanism and a release of catecholamines leading to hypertension and hyperpyrexia may be precipitated by the combination of MAOIs and tyramine-containing foodstuffs and drinks such as mature cheeses, meat extracts and Chianti.

Cough mixtures or nasal decongestants, which contain sympathomimetic agents such as ephedrine, phenylephrine or phenylpropanolamine, are also contraindicated in patients on MAOIs.

Pethidine can interact with MAOIs for reasons which are unclear, and morphine is safer. MAOIs may increase the effects of hypoglycaemic agents so that unexpected falls in blood glucose may occur in diabetics given these antidepressants.

Treatment of a hypertensive crisis is by slow administration of phentolamine 5 mg i.v. at intervals, and tepid sponging and i.m. chlorpromazine to lower temperature. Muscle relaxation with suxamethonium may be required for muscle spasms.

180 B C

Thioridazine has a *piperidine* side chain. Trifluoperazine and fluphenazine have piperazine side chains, while chlorpromazine is an aliphatic compound.

Extrapyramidal effects, hypersensitivity, jaundice, photosensitivity and hypotension are all less common with thioridazine than chlorpromazine. However, pigmentary retinopathy is a particular risk with thioridazine.

Phenothiazines as a group have the property of dopamine receptor blockade, and many of their effects, therapeutic and adverse, are attributable to this. Thioridazine does not *differ* from chlorpromazine in this respect.

181 The following statements concerning electroconvulsive therapy (ECT) are true:
A ECT produces generalized delta activity on the electroencephalograph (EEG)
B for unilateral ECT, the stimulus should be to the dominant hemisphere
C ECT is less effective in people over 70 years old
D the EEG does not return to normal until at least four months after the last treatment
E in depression a standard course of six ECT treatments should be given

182 The following statements concerning tricyclic antidepressants are true:
A trimipramine is relatively sedative
B if antidepressant effect is not seen after seven days, a different antidepressant should be tried
C dothiepin is an example with only mild anticholinergic effects
D they block re-uptake of monoamines into the presynaptic neuron
E some newer antidepressants have been shown to be more effective than amitriptyline

181 A

Patients receiving ECT develop diffuse showing (delta activity) on the EEG. A minority also develop spike foci. In most patients the EEG has returned to normal within three months of ECT.

For unilateral ECT both electrodes should be placed over the non-dominant hemisphere. Dominant unilateral ECT has no advantages and may produce greater memory disturbance than bilateral ECT.

The number of treatments required to relieve depressive symptoms varies considerably from patient to patient, so that a standard course of any set number of treatments should not be adhered to, and the patient's condition should be monitored after each treatment.

On available evidence the efficacy of ECT seems to be at least as good in old age as in younger people.

182 A C D

The effect of tricyclic antidepressants is generally attributed to blockade of re-uptake of neurotransmitter into the presynaptic neuron, as a result of which more neurotransmitter remains in the synaptic cleft, available to activate postsynaptic receptors. The monoamines, noradrenaline and 5-hydroxytryptamine and to a lesser degree dopamine have been implicated in the action of tricyclics.

Of the tricyclic antidepressants, amitriptyline and trimipramine are relatively sedative, while clomipramine, protriptyline and desipramine are less sedative.

Therapeutic effects of a tricyclic antidepressant may not be seen for 14 days so that administration should generally be for at least this time before a different drug is tried.

Since the introduction of imipramine and amitriptyline in the 1950s, other antidepressants have become available, including the tetracyclic compounds mianserin and maprotiline. None, however, is more effective in the alleviation of depression than amitriptyline, and some may be less effective.

183 The following benzodiazepines undergo oxidative metabolism in the liver:
A nitrazepam
B oxazepam
C clobazam
D lorazepam
E diazepam

184 Anticholinergic agents are effective treatment in the following:
A akathisia
B Parkinson's disease
C tardive dyskinesia
D dystonic reactions
E neuroleptic-induced Parkinsonism

183 *A C E*

All the benzodiazepines presently available in the UK except temazepam (Euhypnos, Euhypnos Forte, Normison), oxazepam (Serenid D, Serenid Forte) and lorazepam (Ativan) undergo oxidative metabolism in the liver.

There is a particular risk of hangover effects and accumulation of those benzodiazepines which undergo hepatic oxidation in the elderly and in others with impaired hepatic function.

Another consideration in alcoholics is that acute alcohol intake may inhibit the metabolism of benzodiazepines, excepting probably those which do not undergo hepatic oxidative metabolism.

Hence there is at least a theoretical advantage in using temazepam, oxazepam or lorazepam if required in alcoholics or others with impaired hepatic function.

Hockings N. & Ballinger B.R. (1983) Hypnotics and anxiolytics. *Br. Med. J.* **286**, 1949–51.

184 *B D E*

Extrapyramidal side-effects of neuroleptic drugs are of four kinds:
1 Parkinsonism, which includes rigidity, tremor and hypokinesia.
2 Akathisia—a motor restlessness, usually affecting the legs, which is unpleasant to the patient.
3 Dystonic reactions, which consist of muscle spasms affecting the head and neck usually, although opisthotonus can result. Oculogyric crises may also occur.
4 Tardive dyskinesia (see Question 185).

Parkinson's disease arises as a consequence of degenerative changes, associated with dopamine depletion, in the nigrostriatal pathway. Neuroleptic drugs may produce a similar clinical picture by blockade of dopamine receptors.

It appears that the effects of dopamine in the nigrostriatal pathway are opposed by acetylcholine. Certainly, anticholinergic agents are of value in Parkinsonism (including Parkinson's disease and drug-induced).

L-dopa is not effective in drug-induced Parkinsonism and may induce or exacerbate psychiatric symptoms. Anticholinergic agents are also effective in dystonic reactions, but are of no benefit in akathisia or tardive dyskinesia, and may make this latter condition worse. A benzodiazepine, such as diazepam, is probably more helpful in akathisia.

185 The following may be effective in reducing the severity of tardive dyskinesia in the short-term:
A reserpine
B increasing the dose of neuroleptic
C anticholinergic drugs
D alpha-methyldopa
E tetrabenazene

186 The following are recognized side-effects of electroconvulsive therapy (ECT):
A headache
B diplopia
C muscle aches and pains
D memory disturbance
E confusion

187 The following are recognized features of benzodiazepine medication:
A nasal and conjunctival irritation
B physical dependence
C gastric irritation
D release of aggression
E lethal overdosage

185 A B D E

Tardive dyskinesia characteristically consists of rhythmical movements involving the mouth, tongue and lips, the so-called bucco-lingual masticatory syndrome. Grimacing, lip smacking and tongue protrusion are usual. Less often trunk rocking and choreiform movements in the limbs occur.

Sometimes irreversible, it is associated with prolonged neuroleptic medication and appears to be more common in the old and the brain damaged. The mechanism may be hypersensitivity of dopaminergic receptors.

While drugs which produce dopamine depletion in the brain, such as tetrabenazine, reserpine and alpha-methyldopa, may be of benefit, anticholinergic drugs are not effective, and indeed may make the condition worse.

In the short-term increasing the dose of neuroleptics may afford relief. Withdrawal of neuroleptics may cause initial exacerbation, but this is the best hope of true cure.

186 A C D E

Commonly reported immediate side-effects of ECT include headache, confusion, memory disturbance and muscle pains.

Diplopia is not a recognized side-effect.

187 B D

A physical withdrawal syndrome with benzodiazepines has been reported in some patients after only two months of therapeutic doses. The main symptoms are anxiety, depression insomnia, nausea, depersonalization and perceptual alteration such as noise intolerance.

Release of aggressive behaviour by these drugs has been described. Also precipitation or aggravation of mental confusion particularly in the elderly can occur.

There have been apparently no reported cases of death after oral benzodiazepine overdosage in otherwise healthy subjects.

Gastric irritation is a side-effect of chloral hydrate while chlormethiazole may cause nasal and conjunctival irritation which usually subsides with continued medication.

188 The following antidepressants preferentially inhibit the re-uptake of 5-hydroxytryptamine (5-HT) into the presynaptic neuron:
  A clomipramine
  B imipramine
  C maprotiline
  D desipramine
  E amitriptyline

188 A B E

Amitriptyline, imipramine and clomipramine are tertiary amine tricyclic antidepressants (TCAs) and are metabolized to nortriptyline, desipramine and chlordesipramine respectively (so-called secondary amine TCAs).

Generally, tertiary amine TCAs selectively inhibit the re-uptake of 5-HT through the presynaptic membrane while their secondary amine derivatives inhibit preferentially noradrenaline (NA) re-uptake.

Of the more recently introduced antidepressants trazadone is a predominantly 5-HT re-uptake inhibitor while maprotiline is a relatively pure inhibitor of NA re-uptake. Nomifensine inhibits re-uptake of NA and to a lesser extent 5-HT but, in addition, powerfully inhibits dopamine re-uptake.

Further reading

Clare A. (1980) Electroconvulsive therapy. Psychosurgery. In Clare A. (ed.) *Psychiatry in Dissent: Controversial Issues in Thought and Practice.* 2nd edn. pp. 229–340. London, Tavistock Publications.
Freeman C.P.L. (1979) Electroconvulsive therapy: its current clinical use. *Br. J. Hosp. Med.* **21,** 281.
Hockings N. & Ballinger B.R. (1983) Hypnotics and anxiolytics. *Br. Med. J.* **286,** 1949–51.
Johnson D.A.W. (1981) Practical considerations in the use of depot neuroleptics for the treatment of schizophrenia. In Crown S. (ed.) *Practical Psychiatry.* Vol. 1. pp. 148–54. London, Northwood Publications.
Kendell R.E. (1981) The present status of electroconvulsive therapy. *Br. J. Psychiat.* **139,** 265–84.
Kennedy R.I. (1978) Physical methods of treatment. In Forrest A.D., Affleck J.W. & Zealley A.K. (eds) *Companion to Psychiatric Studies.* 2nd edn. Edinburgh, Churchill Livingstone.
Montgomery S. (1982) Antidepressant drugs. In Granville-Grossman K. (ed.) *Recent Advances in Clinical Psychiatry—4.* pp. 261–79. Edinburgh, Churchill Livingstone.

Psychological Methods of Treatment

189 The following statements concerning psychotherapy are true:
  A resistance refers to opposition to change in psychotherapy
  B meta-analysis provides information on the magnitude of the effect of psychotherapy
  C supportive psychotherapy aims to bring about personality change in the patient
  D counter-transference refers to the patient's attitude towards the therapist
  E Eysenck has claimed that psychoanalytically based therapies are no more effective than spontaneous remission

190 Match each of the following people (A–E) with the most appropriate concept (1–5):
  A Adler
  B Reich
  C Klein
  D Jung
  E Winnicott

  1 paranoid-schizoid position
  2 inferiority complex
  3 transitional object
  4 character armour
  5 extraversion

189 A B E

Resistance is indeed opposition to psychotherapeutic change; in psychoanalytic parlance it is opposition to the process of making the unconscious process conscious.

Transference is the process by which a patient displaces on to his therapist feelings which derive from earlier figures in his life, such as parents. The word may more loosely refer to the patient's attitude toward his therapist. *Counter-transference* refers to the therapist's transference on his patient—the emotions and thoughts which the therapist has about his patient.

While *insight or dynamic psychotherapy* may aim to disrupt a patient's habitual pattern of mental defences and bring about a basic change in his personality, by means including interpretation of transference, the aims of *supportive or superficial psychotherapy* are less radical. Aspects of supportive psychotherapy include changing if possible the patient's social environment, facilitating release of emotion (catharsis), intellectual guidance, bolstering up adaptive defence mechanisms and the relief of emotional distress.

Meta-analysis has been hailed by some as a major breakthrough in psychotherapy research because it permits measurement of the magnitude of any change brought about by psychotherapy. Meta-analysts apply a statistic called the effect size (ES) which is the mean difference between the treated and the control subjects divided by the standard deviation of the control group. ES may be calculated for any outcome measure the researcher chooses to measure, so that meta-analysis may provide a comparative measure of outcome for different therapist or treatment variables in qualitative as well as quantitative terms.

Eysenck's claims on the non-effectiveness of psychoanalytically based therapies have been challenged by Bergin (1971).

Bergin A.E. (1971) The evaluation of therapeutic outcomes. In Bergin A.E. & Garfield S.L. (eds) *Handbook of Psychotherapy and Behaviour Change*. 1st edn. New York, John Wiley & Sons.
Crown S. (1981) Psychotherapy research today. *Br. J. Hosp. Med.* **25,** 492–503.
Eysenck H.J. (1965) The effects of psychotherapy. *Int. J. Psychiat.* **1,** 97–178.

190 A2 B4 C1 D5 E3

See Question 191.

191 Match each of the following people (A–E) with the associated concept (1–5):
A Jung
B Klein
C Adler
D Winnicott
E Reich

1 play analysis
2 striving for power
3 orgone energy
4 good enough mother
5 archetype

191 A5 B1 C2 D4 E3

Jung described three levels to the psyche—consciousness, the personal unconscious and the collective unconscious. It is the collective unconscious which contains the collective myths of the race to which the individual belongs. Its deepest level is the universal unconscious, a stratum common to mankind and indeed also to his primate and animal ancestry. Jung described *archetypes* such as the Great Mother and the Great Father of All, which he regarded as recurrent themes deriving from the collective unconscious. His conceptualization of personality was of an outer part in contact with the world called the *persona* and that people are predominantly either *extravert* or introvert in the way in which they interact with reality. Underlying the *persona* of conscious life is the unconscious female image in men (*anima*) and the unconscious male image in women (*animus*).

Adler differed from Freud in his greater emphasis on power as a motivational drive. According to him feelings of inferiority (*inferiority complex*) which were sometimes based on actual physical handicap ('organ inferiority') led to a compensatory *striving for power*.

Reich pursued a line of thought begun by Freud that undischarged libido is converted into anxiety. Later he appears to have believed that a life force, which he called *orgone energy*, 'bio-energy' or 'primordial cosmic energy' could not only be experimentally demonstrated but could be stored in 'orgone boxes' or 'orgone energy accumulators'. A further theory was that body tensions (*character armour*) could reflect habitual emotional states.

Melanie Klein and Anna Freud pioneered child analysis. While Anna Freud's methods were adapted from techniques of adult psychoanalysis and were applicable to children old enough to cooperate and with a sufficient verbal capacity, Melanie Klein *analysed the play* of children as young as two years old. She drew attention to so-called primitive defence mechanisms such as projection, splitting and introjection and described the *paranoid-schizoid* and depressive positions.

Winnicott introduced the concept of the *good enough mother* and also the concept of the *transitional object*—an object such as a doll which the subject regards as part of the way between himself and another person.

Segal H. (1964) *Introduction to the Works of Melanie Klein*. London, Heinemann Medical Books.

Winnicott D.W. (1974) *Playing and Reality*. Harmondsworth, Penguin Books.

192 The following people are associated with particular theoretical schools or therapies. Match each person (A–F) with the most appropriate school or therapy (1–6):
A Freud
B Main
C Perls
D Adler
E Fairbairn
F Jung

1 Individual Psychology
2 Object Relations Theory
3 Psychoanalysis
4 Gestalt Therapy
5 Analytical Psychology
6 Therapeutic Community

192 A3 B6 C4 D1 E2 F5

Psychoanalysis refers to a theoretical framework founded by Freud and to the method of psychotherapy based on it. Arguably all other forms of dynamic psychotherapy stem from psychoanalysis.

Jung and Adler branched away from Freud to form their own schools of *Analytical Psychology* and *Individual Psychology* respectively (see Question 191).

A more recent thread in psychoanalytic thinking has been *Object Relations Theory* developed by Fairburn, Guntrip, Winnicott and Balint. Central to this theory is the individual's need to relate to objects; this is seen as a fundamental drive in man. Incidentally, the word 'object' is not used here in the sense of an inanimate thing. In the context of psychoanalytical writing objects are actual or symbolic representations of persons or parts of persons.

Perls who developed *Gestalt Therapy* considered neurosis to be due to splitting in the 'wholes' or *Gestalten* which unify mind and body and a person and his environment. The mode of therapy derived from this conceptual framework is usually carried out in a group and aims at immediacy of experience and awareness. The focus is on present feelings and thoughts, and directness of expression.

Therapeutic Community is a term first used by Main. It has been used in different ways, but in the sense of the therapeutic milieu described by Maxwell Jones it refers to a setting in which hierarchies of authority are eschewed and communal living based on principles of permissiveness and democratic decision-making aim to promote individual responsibility, interpersonal skills and more acceptable social behaviour.

Jones M. (1968) *Social Psychiatry in Practice: The Idea of the Therapeutic Community*. Harmondsworth, Penguin Books.

Main T.F. (1946) The hospital as a therapeutic institution. *Bull. Menninger Clin.* **10**, 66–70.

193 The following are non-specific factors (or common therapeutic factors) in psychotherapy:
  A promotion of hope
  B facilitation of emotional arousal
  C 'flooding'
  D interpretation of the transference neurosis
  E the therapist–patient relationship

193 *A B E*

The term 'non-specific factor' may be used in different ways, but perhaps most often refers to an aspect of therapy which is not unique to any particular therapy but is common to many forms of treatment. An obvious example is the therapist–patient relationship.

Frank *et al.* (1978) have considered the following to be non-specific factors in psychotherapy: arousal of hope, the provision of an explanatory myth or mental model for the patient's problems and their treatment, the acquisition by the patient of knowledge concerning the origins of his problems and alternative means of dealing with them, the facilitation of emotional arousal, the provision of experiences of success which increase the patient's sense of mastery over his environment and an intense, confiding relationship with the therapist.

Interpretation of the transference neurosis is a specific ingredient of psychoanalytically based therapy, while flooding is a mode of behaviour therapy used to treat phobias.

Frank J.D., Hoehn-Sarik R., Imber S.D., Liberman B.L. & Stone A.R. (1978) *Effective Ingredients of Successful Psychotherapy.* New York, Brunner-Mazel.

194 For each therapy (1–5) select the person (A–E) who is associated with it:
A Rogers
B Ellis
C Berne
D Moreno
E Janov

1 Transactional Analysis
2 Client-Centred Psychotherapy
3 Psychodrama
4 Primal Therapy
5 Rational Emotive Therapy

A2 B5 C1 D3 E4

Moreno was the originator of *psychodrama*; (he probably also coined the term 'group psychotherapy'). He related neurosis to a failure in the expression of emotion and advocated role play and the re-enactment by patients of their problems. In psychodrama the therapist directs the proceedings and a stage may be used to enhance the theatrical effect.

Janov traced the origins of neurosis back to the pain of birth trauma. He proposed that *Primal Therapy*, in encouraging the discharge of emotion in screaming, enabled the release of this pent-up pain.

Eric Berne's mode of psychotherapy called *Transactional Analysis* is based on a model of personality which assumes three states of function—those of parent, adult and child. This corresponds roughly to Freud's structural model of the mind consisting of super-ego, ego and id. Berne has looked at the ways in which people interact in terms of 'games'. His terminology, in using familiar words, may arguably convey meaning to more people.

Carl Rogers advocated the non-directive techniques of *Client-Centred Psychotherapy*. He proposed that a person is capable of growth and self-fulfilment given the opportunity provided by an 'enabling' relationship. Non-possessive warmth, genuineness and empathy in the therapist are considered to be necessary and sufficient conditions for effective therapy.

Rational Emotive Therapy of Ellis involves directly challenging a patient's unhelpful ideas and attitudes. The therapist uses argument in attacking the patient's irrational belief system. This therapy assumes that behavioural change will ensue from a shift in the patient's cognitive position.

Berne E. (1964) *Games People Play*. New York, Grove Press.
Rogers C.R. (1951) *Client Centred Psychotherapy*. Boston, Houghton-Mifflin.

195 According to Freud, unconscious mental contents become manifest in
  A dreams
  B neurotic symptoms
  C the *anima*
  D bio-energy
  E parapraxes

195 *A B E*

Freudian theory holds that unconscious mental material may become manifest or conscious as *dreams, neurotic symptoms, parapraxes,* by free association, and under the influence of drugs, alcohol or hypnosis.

Freud drew a distinction between the manifest content of a *dream* (the dream, as recalled after sleep) and the latent content (its meaning as revealed by interpretation using the technique of free association). He theorized that the latent content is transformed by the processes of condensation, displacement, plastic representation, and fixed symbolism, into the manifest content. This 'dreamwork' accomplishes censorship of content shocking to the ego and so permits sleep to continue.

Parapraxes are erroneous actions caused by the interference of unconscious mental processes. Slips of the tongue are examples of these Freudian slips.

Bio-energy is a concept of Wilhelm Reich and the *anima* is Jung's term for the unconscious female image in men (see Question 191).

Freud S. (1901) *The Psychopathology of Everyday Life.* Standard edn. Vol. 6. London, Hogarth Press, 1960.

196 Match each of the following people (A–E) with the associated concept (1–5):
A Yalom
B Seligman
C Bion
D Minuchin
E Beck

1 basic assumptions
2 logical systematic errors
3 family structure
4 curative factors
5 learned helplessness

196 A4 B5 C1 D3 E2

Minuchin considers the *structure of families* in terms of subsystems—for instance, parental and sibling subsystems. Problems arise in a family either when boundaries between subsystems are not sufficiently defined and family members are enmeshed together, or when the converse situation exists and each family member constitutes a different subsystem and the family is fragmented.

Yalom has described certain *curative factors*, or factors which are capable of producing beneficial change, in group therapy. These include universality, altruism, instillation of hope, corrective recapitulation of the primary family group, interpersonal learning, imitative behaviour and group cohesiveness.

Bion described unconscious, emotional forces influencing the working of a group, which he called *basic assumptions*. These are dependency—an expectation that the group leader will provide solutions to all problems, fight-flight—an assumption that the group is threatened, which results in emotions of fear and hostility, and pairing—an assumption that a new leader will arise.

Beck considers that a depressed person has a cognitive triad of negative attitudes regarding himself, the present and the future. So-called *logical systematic errors* in thinking, examples of which are arbitrary inference, selective abstraction, over-generalization and minimization or magnification, lead to faulty conclusions. In cognitive therapy for depression Beck advocates that the patient's depressive ideation is pinpointed, its validity challenged and alternative self-statements substituted in a process of cognitive restructuring. Reality testing should be used to reinforce the conviction that certain beliefs are invalid and also to test out alternative, more adaptive beliefs.

Seligman, from results of animal studies, related human depression to *learned helplessness*—a situation thought to arise when a person believes that his actions have no control over his experience of pain or pleasure (when reward or punishment is non-contingent on action). Animals subjected to repeated unpleasant stimuli which they could not avoid, showed passivity, retarded learning, undereating and lack of aggressiveness—features similar to the symptoms of human depression.

Beck A.T. (1967) *Depression: Clinical, Experimental and Theoretical Aspects*. London, Staples Press.
Bion W.R. (1961) *Experience in Groups*. London, Tavistock Publications.
Minuchin S. (1977) *Families and Family Therapy*. London, Tavistock Publications.
Seligman M.E.P. (1975) *Helplessness*. San Francisco, W.H. Freeman & Company.
Yalom I.D. (1970) *Theory and Practice of Group Psychotherapy*. New York, Basic Books.

197 Match each of the following people (A–E) with the most appropriate treatment method (1–5):
A   Crowe
B   Ayllon and Azrin
C   Meyer
D   Cautela
E   Argyle

1   social skills training
2   apotrepic therapy
3   covert sensitization
4   contract marital therapy
5   token economy

197 A4 B5 C2 D3 E1

Token economy based on operant conditioning theory was pioneered by Ayllon and Azrin and has been used to promote rehabilitation and self-care in the chronically institutionalized as well as chronic schizophrenics. Tokens given as immediate reward for appropriate behaviour may later be 'cashed in' for reinforcers such as money or time watching television. Although a potent means of modifying behaviour, there may be difficulties in the maintenance of the desired behaviour and its generalization to other situations.

Argyle attempted to delineate the elements, verbal and non-verbal, which constitute appropriate social interaction and communication. In conversation these include picking up cues from the other person and modifying one's own performance accordingly. A type of treatment for socially inadequate patients—*social skills training*—has been derived from this. It is often carried out with a group of patients and involves role-play or rehearsal of particular social situations. Video recording can provide feedback on the patient's performance.

Crowe has described a technique of *marital therapy* based on a reciprocity or 'give to get' principle, whereby one partner undertakes to change his behaviour as requested by the other, in exchange for modifications in his spouse's behaviour which he desires.

In *covert sensitization* described by Cautela, covert or mental events act as negative reinforcers. This method has been used in the treatment of obsessions and sexual deviation and involves the patient first imagining, as clearly as possible, the circumstances of the undesired behaviour and then the therapist suggesting to him he is experiencing some unpleasant sensation, such as nausea.

Meyer has described the use of *apotrepic therapy* for obsessional rituals (see Question 200).

198 The following are true of operant conditioning:
A reinforcement precedes and elicits the response
B continuous (rather than partial) reinforcement leads to a response which is more resistant to extinction
C it is sometimes called 'instrumental learning'
D reinforcement increases the chance that a stimulus will in future evoke a response
E extinction is a permanent state

198 C D

Operant conditioning, sometimes termed 'instrumental learning', involves changing the frequency of spontaneous behaviour by reward or punishment.

In classical conditioning reinforcement is the unconditioned stimulus, which precedes and elicits the response. In operant conditioning, however, reinforcement follows the response.

Reinforcement by definition is that event which increases the probability that a stimulus will in future evoke a response. It may be either continuous or partial. In continuous reinforcement every appropriate response is reinforced. Partial or intermittent reinforcement is when only a proportion of correct responses is reinforced and results in learning which is more resistant to extinction.

Extinction refers to the tendency of learned responses to disappear, if reinforcement is withdrawn. It is not a permanent state of affairs, however, and responses tend to recur—the phenomenon of 'spontaneous recovery'.

199 The following names of people are associated with certain theoretical concepts. Match each person (A–E) with the most appropriate concept (1–5):
A Mowrer
B Skinner
C Bandura
D Seligman
E Pavlov

1 modelling
2 classical conditioning
3 two-stage theory of fear and avoidance
4 operant conditioning
5 preparedness

199 A3 B4 C1 D5 E2

Classical conditioning refers to the formation of an association between a conditioned stimulus (CS) and a response through the repeated presentation of the CS in a controlled relationship with an unconditioned stimulus (US) that originally elicits that response. This was first described by Pavlov and in his early experiments using dogs, food was the US and salivation the unconditioned response (UR). After repeated pairing of a bell ringing with food placed in the dog's mouth it was found that the bell ringing (CS) on its own elicited salivation (now the conditioned response, CR).

Skinner described *operant conditioning* (see Question 198). The *two-stage theory of fear and avoidance* of Mowrer involves both classical and operant conditioning principles. It provides an explanation for the formation of phobias. In the first stage by pairing a neutral stimulus with a stimulus which normally elicits fear, the former will eventually evoke fear on its own. The fear acts as a negative reinforcer, so that any act of avoidance in preventing or reducing the fear will tend to be repeated.

The induction of a fear of white rats in Little Albert (see Question 74) could be interpreted using the two-stage theory as follows:

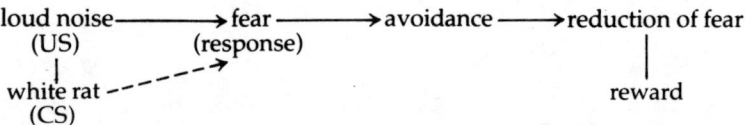

It is interesting that certain stimuli such as writhing or darting animals and heights seem to have an increased potential to elicit fear reactions, compared to say guns, which actually present more risk. Seligman has referred to this enhanced potential as *preparedness*.

A type of learning which occurs by observation of another person's behaviour has been termed *modelling* by Bandura, e.g. people becoming less likely to break the law after observing others punished for law breaking. Quite complex behaviour, such as social behaviour, may be learnt vicariously in this way.

200 The following are recognized techniques in the treatment of obsessional cleaning rituals associated with a phobia of contamination:
  A drug-assisted abreaction
  B thought withdrawal
  C response prevention
  D modelling
  E exposure to the source of feared contamination

200 C D E

Techniques used in the therapy of obsessional rituals include *exposing* the patient to the fear situation while at the same time restraining him usually by verbal means from carrying out any rituals (*response prevention*). *Modelling*, whereby the patient either merely observes the therapist in contact with the feared situation (passive modelling) or is encouraged to imitate him (participant modelling), is normally an additional factor in the treatment programme.

Meyer termed a treatment programme for obsessions, involving exposure and response prevention, *apotrepic treatment* after the Greek word *apotrepos*, to turn away or dissuade.

Drug-assisted abreaction is not a recognized treatment for obsessional rituals and thought withdrawal is a passivity experience—an experience that thoughts are being taken out of the mind by an external force.

Further reading

Barker P. (1981) *Basic Family Therapy*. London, Granada.
Bebbington P. (1979) Behaviour therapy. In Hill P., Murray R. & Thorley A. (eds) *Essentials of Postgraduate Psychiatry*. pp. 683–702. London, Academic Press.
Bloch S. (ed.) (1979) *An Introduction to the Psychotherapies*. Oxford, Oxford University Press.
Bloch S. (1982) Psychotherapy. In Granville-Grossman K. (ed.) *Recent Advances in Clinical Psychiatry*—4. pp. 25–45. Edinburgh, Churchill Livingstone.
Brown D. & Pedder J. (1979) *Introduction to Psychotherapy*. London, Tavistock Publications.
Brown J.A.C. (1961) *Freud and the Post-freudians*. Harmondsworth, Penguin Books.
Clark R.W. (1982) *Freud. The Man and the Cause*. London, Granada.
Marks I.M. (1981) Psychiatry and behavioural psychotherapy. *Br. J. Psychiat.* **139**, 74.